Childhood Epilepsy: Management from Diagnosis to Remission

Childhood Epilepsy: Management from Diagnosis to Remission

Edited by

Richard Appleton

Consultant Pediatric Neurologist, The Roald Dahl EEG Unit, Pediatric Neurosciences Foundation, Alder Hey Children's Hospital NHS Foundation Trust, Liverpool, and Clinical Lecturer, University of Liverpool, UK

Peter Camfield

Professor Emeritus, Department of Pediatrics, Dalhousie University and the IWK Health Center, Halifax, Nova Scotia, Canada

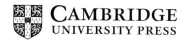

CAMBRIDGE
UNIVERSITY PRESS

CAMBRIDGE UNIVERSITY PRESS

Cambridge, New York, Melbourne, Madrid, Cape Town,
Singapore, São Paulo, Delhi, Tokyo, Mexico City

Cambridge University Press
The Edinburgh Building, Cambridge CB2 8RU, UK

Published in the United States of America by Cambridge University Press, New York

www.cambridge.org
Information on this title: www.cambridge.org/9780521763257

First published 2011

Printed in the United Kingdom at the University Press, Cambridge

A catalog record for this publication is available from the British Library

Library of Congress Cataloging in Publication Data

Childhood epilepsy : from diagnosis to remission / edited by Richard Appleton, Peter Camfield.
      p. ; cm.
   Includes bibliographical references and index.
   ISBN 978-0-521-76325-7 (Paperback)
1. Epilepsy in children.   I. Appleton, Richard   II. Camfield, Peter   III. Title.
   [DNLM: 1. Epilepsy.   2. Child. WL 385]
   RJ496.E6C462 2011
   618.92′853–dc22

                                                                                    2011001411

ISBN 978-0-521-76325-7 Paperback

Every effort has been made in preparing this book to provide accurate and
up-to-date information which is in accord with accepted standards and
practice at the time of publication. Although case histories are drawn from
actual cases, every effort has been made to disguise the identities of the
individuals involved. Nevertheless, the authors, editors and publishers can
make no warranties that the information contained herein is totally free
from error, not least because clinical standards are constantly changing
through research and regulation. The authors, editors and publishers
therefore disclaim all liability for direct or consequential damages
resulting from the use of material contained in this book. Readers are
strongly advised to pay careful attention to information provided by the
manufacturer of any drugs or equipment that they plan to use.

Contents

Preface   *page* vii
List of contributors   viii

1.   The only place to start: making the diagnosis of epilepsy   1
     Peter Camfield and Richard Appleton

2.   Epilepsy beginning in infancy   5
     Stewart Macleod and Elaine Wyllie

3.   Epilepsy beginning in middle childhood   29
     Elaine Wirrell and John H. Livingston

4.   Epilepsy beginning in adolescence   73
     Tim Martland and Carol Camfield

5.   Risks and hazards of epilepsy   108
     Ingrid Tuxhorn and J. Helen Cross

6.   Status epilepticus   126
     Richard Appleton and Peter Camfield

7.   The prevention of epilepsy and its consequences   133
     Richard Appleton and Peter Camfield

8.   Medico-legal aspects of epilepsy   139
     Richard Appleton and Peter Camfield

Glossary   143
Index   150

Preface

This is a short, practical and unique textbook about children with epilepsy. The book focuses on the evolution of the disorder from diagnosis to either remission or ongoing care into adult life. Some children will outgrow their seizures and discontinuation of antiepileptic medication will be entirely appropriate while others will require lifelong treatment and support. The book addresses important diagnostic and investigative decisions and associated co-morbid problems, and discusses both the specific antiepileptic treatment as well as the holistic management of childhood epilepsy.

The book uses a novel approach and approaches epilepsy as it develops chronologically, beginning in infancy and progressing through mid-childhood into adolescence, and with a common framework, namely the natural history from diagnosis to remission or chronicity.

Finally, we have emphasized that epilepsy syndrome diagnosis is often critical for long-term care and the honest and realistic counseling for the family. In doing so, we hope that we have accurately represented what most clinicians face in their seizure or epilepsy clinics, week after week.

We believe that it will meet a clear demand for a book that is specifically designed for the general pediatrician who has a specific interest and responsibility for delivering comprehensive care for children with epilepsy.

In reviewing previous publications and in designing the scope of this book, we also identified specific topics not previously addressed but considered to be important and useful. We have therefore included chapters on the 'Risks and hazards of epilepsy,' 'Prevention of epilepsy and its consequences' and 'Medico-legal aspects of epilepsy.' We have also included a brief, overview chapter on 'Status epilepticus' and a glossary.

Each chapter has been written enthusiastically and jointly by specialists in epilepsy in Great Britain and North America, who collectively have over a century of experience in managing childhood epilepsy in both secondary and tertiary care.

Throughout the book we have strived to write a comprehensive and, above all, practical book for the many general pediatricians engaged in the care of children with epilepsy.

Contributors

Richard Appleton
Consultant Pediatric Neurologist, The Roald Dahl EEG Unit, Pediatric
Neurosciences Foundation, Alder Hey Children's Hospital NHS Foundation Trust,
Liverpool, and Clinical Lecturer, University of Liverpool, UK

Carol Camfield
Professor Emeritus, Department of Pediatrics, Dalhousie University and Department
of Pediatric Neurology and the IWK Health Center, Halifax, Nova Scotia, Canada

Peter Camfield
Professor Emeritus, Department of Pediatrics, Dalhousie University and the IWK
Health Center, Halifax, Nova Scotia, Canada

J. Helen Cross
The Prince of Wales' Chair of Childhood Epilepsy, UCL – Institute of Child
Health, Great Ormond Street Hospital for Children NHS Trust, London and the
National Centre for Young People with Epilepsy, Neurosciences Unit,
The Wolfson Centre, London, UK

John H. Livingston
Department of Pediatric Neurology, The Leeds Teaching Hospitals NHS Trust,
Leeds, UK

Stewart Macleod
Consultant Pediatric Neurologist, Fraser of Allander Neurosciences Unit,
Royal Hospital for Sick Children, Glasgow, UK

Tim Martland
Consultant Pediatric Neurologist, Royal Manchester Children's Hospital,
Pendlebury, Manchester, UK

Ingrid Tuxhorn
Professor, Department of Pediatrics, Case Western Reserve University, Chief,
Division of Pediatric Epilepsy, Rainbow Babies and Children's University Hospital,
Cleveland, OH, USA

Elaine Wirrell
Professor of Neurology, Division of Child and Adolescent Neurology, Mayo Clinic, Rochester, MN, USA

Elaine Wyllie
Director, Center for Pediatric Neurology, Cleveland Clinic Foundation, Cleveland, OH, USA

The only place to start: making the diagnosis of epilepsy

Peter Camfield and Richard Appleton

Epilepsy is defined as the tendency for recurrent seizures to occur without acute provocation. Every child's (and adult's) brain is capable of generating a seizure with certain pro-convulsive drugs and it should therefore be of no surprise that seizures may be provoked by numerous other factors including: an acute metabolic (biochemical) disturbance, central nervous infection, drug intoxication or acute head trauma. The risk of epilepsy developing after acute and provoked (symptomatic) seizures is low (3–5%) and therefore the occurrence of acute seizures cannot contribute to, and should not influence, the diagnosis of epilepsy. Emotional stress is not considered to be a provoking factor.

Epilepsy has protean manifestations. Some children present with generalized tonic-clonic seizures (convulsions), while others present with staring spells (usually absence seizures), periods of confusion with or without automatisms (usually complex partial [focal] seizures), limb or body jerks (myoclonus), spasms (infantile or epileptic spasms), falls or drops (usually atonic or astatic but also tonic seizures), loss of speech and social interactions and/or cognitive function (Landau–Kleffner syndrome), and variants of paroxysmal events during sleep (often frontal lobe or, less commonly, temporal lobe seizures).

Epilepsy and some epilepsy syndromes may be diagnosed relatively quickly after a few tonic-clonic seizures (as these are usually dramatic and understandably frighten the family). Conversely, other syndromes may be diagnosed after some considerable time and only after the child has experienced a number of seizures. This is often because infrequent or only subtle seizures usually do not prompt parents to seek medical advice. Once seizures have been seen to occur very frequently, and specifically absence or myoclonic seizures, the diagnosis may be more straightforward; however, when patients present with only a few seizures the

Childhood Epilepsy: Management from Diagnosis to Remission, ed. Richard Appleton and Peter Camfield. Published by Cambridge University Press. © Cambridge University Press 2011.

diagnosis is more challenging. A common scenario is the child presenting after a first, unprovoked 'major seizure,' i.e., a generalized tonic-clonic or prolonged complex partial seizure. After a first unprovoked 'major seizure' the chances of a recurrence are about 50%, and usually within the following six to 12 months. Clearly there are many children who will have an isolated unprovoked seizure and do not have a 'tendency for recurrent seizures'; they should not be diagnosed as having epilepsy, regardless of the results of investigations. However, in many cases the first 'major seizure' is not in fact the first seizure and a careful history may reveal preceding 'minor seizures' (and usually collectively and erroneously termed 'petit mals'), such as myoclonus or absence that had not worried the family sufficiently to prompt them to seek medical advice. If there is a convincing history of 'minor seizures,' alongside a clear history of a first 'major' (tonic-clonic) seizure, then it would be appropriate to make a diagnosis of epilepsy.

If a person has two unprovoked seizures then the chance of further seizures increases significantly to 80–90%, a recurrence risk that justifies the diagnosis of epilepsy. Consequently, the operational diagnosis of epilepsy is usually defined as the occurrence of two or more unprovoked seizures – and irrespective of the seizure type.

The diagnosis of a seizure – and epilepsy – is a clinical diagnosis in nearly all cases. In most situations, most seizures will have stopped long before the child is seen for medical advice. A careful history is the only diagnostic test and there are numerous paroxysmal disorders that may, on only limited 'sound-bites' of a history, mimic epileptic seizures. The most common is the brief, generalized, total body stiffening with or without a few myoclonic or clonic movements that characterizes vasovagal syncope or a reflex anoxic seizure. The clinical history must include where the episodes occurred and at what time, what the child was doing at the time and whether there was any possible provoking factor. For syncope, a typical scenario will be a dentist's surgery, the sight of blood or sudden pain, or in a particularly hot environment. The patient often reports the premonitory symptoms of syncope such as light-headedness and feeling cold and clammy. This is followed by gradual graying and loss of vision. Observers will note extreme pallor with a limp fall and then stiffening with a few body jerks – myoclonic or clonic movements. Thus a history must be obtained from the patient and a witness. Incontinence more commonly occurs during a seizure but also occurs during syncope if the child has not recently urinated. The finding of a carpet burn on the face or a limb and an unexplained bitten tongue, particularly the side of the tongue, is much more suggestive of a generalized tonic-clonic seizure.

There are no investigations that can replace or short-cut the medical history. The results of an electroencephalogram (EEG) may be particularly misleading. If the patient has an actual seizure during the EEG recording then the diagnosis of epilepsy will be confirmed or refuted, in most cases; focal seizures arising from the mesial frontal lobe are an exception and the surface EEG may show no obvious change during or following the seizure. Unfortunately, other than in childhood-onset absence, photosensitive epilepsy or, occasionally, West syndrome a child is unlikely to experience a seizure and the EEG is nearly always undertaken when the patient is well. The hope is to find either focal or generalized 'epileptic discharges' (traditionally defined as spikes, spike and wave, or sharp waves on the EEG). It is important to understand the limitations of the EEG in the diagnosis of epilepsy:

- Approximately 3–5% of 'normal' children who never have experienced, and never will experience, a seizure will show spike activity or spike and slow-wave activity on the EEG.
- Conversely, approximately 20–25% of children with definite epilepsy will show no epileptic discharge on a routine EEG.

Consequently, the finding of epileptic discharges on EEG is neither sufficiently sensitive nor specific to make the diagnosis of epilepsy. Again, the diagnosis can only be achieved by the clinical history. If the history is vague, incomplete or non-diagnostic, we are of the opinion that it is best to defer the diagnosis until there are more obvious epileptic attacks or if additional history, with or without video footage of the episodes, becomes available. There is good evidence that epilepsy is often falsely diagnosed and even pediatric neurologists may occasionally disagree, when the history from frightened or inarticulate parents is unusual or incomplete – or the history has not been obtained from an eye-witness of the episodes. A false diagnosis of epilepsy may result in significant and considerable harm by inducing stigma, exposing the child to potentially dangerous medications, restricting the child's activities and adversely affecting both the child's psyche and that of their family.

The role and the importance of the EEG are not in making the diagnosis of epilepsy but in:

- helping to identify and define the specific epilepsy syndrome
- identifying areas of focal brain dysfunction that will assist the interpretation of brain imaging studies (magnetic resonance imaging [MRI])
- the confirmation (or exclusion) of non-convulsive status epilepticus.

For example, a 'normal' early school-aged child who presents with characteristic focal seizures at night may show the characteristic broad, central EEG spikes or sharp waves that, together with the clinical history, will establish the diagnosis of benign partial epilepsy with centro-temporal spikes (BECTS). However, another 'normal' child of the same age but with a different semiology to their nocturnal seizures and with an EEG that demonstrates discrete frontal spikes and a slow-wave abnormality might have a frontal brain tumor.

An epilepsy syndrome is currently defined on the basis of largely subjective criteria, including:

- the age at onset of the seizures
- the seizure type or types
- the child's neuro-developmental profile
- the EEG (and ideally, both an inter-ictal and ictal recording).

In the future, it is possible, if not likely, that with the identification of specific genetic or biochemical markers, or both, the term 'epilepsy syndrome' may be more appropriately replaced by the term 'epilepsy disease.'

Neuro-imaging, even with MRI, also does not contribute to the diagnosis of epilepsy. An abnormal computed tomography (CT) or MRI scan in a child with uncertain paroxysmal episodes does not necessarily mean that the episodes are epileptic in origin. The role of CT in the investigation of epilepsy is now largely redundant and, in addition, involves unnecessary irradiation that is equivalent to over 100 chest x-rays. Magnetic resonance imaging is far more effective than CT in detecting significant cortical abnormalities that may cause epilepsy and MRI is generally recommended once a child has been diagnosed with a non-benign focal or non-idiopathic generalized epilepsy.

In summary, epilepsy has many manifestations and its correct diagnosis depends on a comprehensive and accurate history obtained from an eye-witness of the child's paroxysmal episodes. Information on the diagnosis, prognosis and management of specific epilepsy syndromes and other, non-syndromic epilepsies requires the additional and specialist knowledge that is illustrated in this book.

2

Epilepsy beginning in infancy

Stewart Macleod and Elaine Wyllie

Introduction

Epilepsy and epileptic seizures are common in infancy. A population-based study of Canadian children found an incidence of epilepsy of 118/100,000 infants aged less than one year (excluding neonates), falling to 42/100,000 in the second year of life (1). Seizures that are considered epileptic are of course even more common. Approximately 3% of all children will have at least one febrile seizure, the majority of which will occur in the first two years of life. Acute symptomatic seizures are also common in this age group with common etiologies including CNS infection, trauma and transient biochemical impairment (e.g., hyponatraemia, hypoglycemia and hypocalcemia). Clearly, evaluation of infants with seizures must always include a careful search for an underlying and potentially treatable cause.

As in any age group, the diagnosis of epilepsy in infants relies on an accurate history and second-by-second and minute-by-minute account of the event as it starts, progresses and ends. It may be easier to obtain good first-hand witness accounts of paroxysmal events in this age group as young infants spend the majority of time with their immediate care-givers. Seizure semiology in infants can be complex:

- Generalized tonic-clonic seizures, although rare in this age group (particularly before the age of one year), should be easy to diagnose.
- Myoclonic seizures may be more difficult to recognize and usually occur in a number of symptomatic and presumed symptomatic epilepsies, often with a metabolic etiology.
- Infantile spasms are usually easily recognized although the seizure semiology is not familiar to parents and primary care clinicians (general practitioners).
- Focal seizures may be particularly difficult to recognize, even by pediatricians with some experience in treating epilepsy.

Childhood Epilepsy: Management from Diagnosis to Remission, ed. Richard Appleton and Peter Camfield. Published by Cambridge University Press. © Cambridge University Press 2011.

Home video recordings can be very useful to fully appreciate subtle motor phenomena including head and/or eye deviation (2). It is always valuable to obtain as detailed a history as possible, including the ante- and peri-natal history, developmental history and specifically whether there is a family history of early infantile seizures. The oldest surviving female family member usually provides the most information when obtaining an accurate family history. The benign idiopathic epilepsies of early infancy are inherited in a dominant fashion (with variable penetrance), making an extended family history invaluable.

The investigative process should not stop with the diagnosis of 'epilepsy.' Whenever possible any underlying epilepsy syndrome should be diagnosed but it is probably more important to try to identify an underlying etiology. An etiology will be found in approximately 70–80% of infants ($<$ 12 months) with symptomatic seizures. These will include structural brain lesions and biochemical abnormalities. Current brain imaging techniques, particularly magnetic resonance imaging (MRI) has increased the number of identified cerebral lesions in this age group. A wide spectrum of abnormalities may be seen, but most are acquired (destructive) or developmental (malformations). Genetic abnormalities are increasingly recognized, ranging from small chromosomal microdeletions to single gene mutation syndromes such as those found in severe myoclonic epilepsy of infancy (SMEI or Dravet syndrome) with mutations in sodium ion channels or GABA-receptor genes. Finally, there are a number of potentially treatable neurological disorders which present at this age with epileptic seizures. There should be a high index of suspicion when considering these conditions; it is important that they be diagnosed as early as possible because early treatment may improve the long-term developmental and cognitive potential.

It is important to emphasize that many epilepsy syndromes which occur in infancy are rare and clinicians may only see one or two cases during their careers.

An important concept that is particularly poignant in epilepsy in infants is the 'epileptic encephalopathy,' or 'catastrophic epilepsy' as termed by other epilepsy specialists. An encephalopathy is any process which disturbs cerebral function. The list of conditions in pediatrics that can cause an encephalopathy is long but by definition an 'epileptic encephalopathy' is a disorder in which the cerebral dysfunction is considered to be primarily caused by the patient's epileptic seizures or frequent paroxysmal EEG abnormalities, rather than the underlying etiology of the epilepsy. The effects of an epileptic encephalopathy may sometimes be permanent with neurological and cognitive deficits persisting even if the seizures are fully controlled. A number of these disorders occur throughout all age ranges. Although each one is rare, collectively they constitute a significant proportion of epilepsy practice. Finally, most of the epileptic encephalopathies present in infancy, including pyridoxine-dependency and Ohtahara, West and Dravet syndromes.

Symptomatic epilepsies in early infancy

Symptomatic epilepsies constitute the majority of cases in this age group, which reflects the large number of symptomatic etiologies which can potentially present with epileptic seizures. Obviously, some of the etiologies can present with epilepsy at any age (e.g., epilepsy associated with congenital hemiplegia or epilepsy as a manifestation of a malformation of cortical development). In contrast, there are many etiologies that invariably present with epileptic seizures in infancy (e.g., the seizures in pyridoxine-dependency, migrating partial seizures [epilepsy] in infancy, and Rett syndrome caused by mutations in the CDKL5 gene).

A comprehensive protocol or guideline-driven approach to the investigation of infantile seizures will help the clinician to undertake the relevant investigations. However, such an approach means that the infant will be subjected to a number of potentially invasive and unpleasant, costly and unnecessary investigations with little chance of identifying the etiology. Consequently, it may be very useful to consider a rational framework or algorithm for the investigation of these infants using the following approach:

- a structural abnormality
- a genetic disorder
- a metabolic disorder.

Obviously, there may be some disorders that overlap with this rather arbitrary classification; this is well illustrated by the tuberous sclerosis complex which has well-defined imaging features on MRI, as well as an identifiable genetic mutation in approximately 80% of children. This overlap is also seen in a large number of metabolic disorders.

Disorders of brain structure

Structural brain lesions are the most common cause of epilepsy in infants. The lesions can be pre-natal (e.g., congenital malformations including cortical dysplasias, neuronal migration abnormalities, or destructive lesions caused by maternally acquired infection), peri-natal (e.g., caused by moderate or severe neonatal hypoxic–ischemic encephalopathy), or post-natally acquired (e.g., caused by meningitis/encephalitis or trauma, or a brain tumor). Brain tumors in infants and young children typically occur in the posterior fossa (cerebellum and brain stem) and present with symptoms and signs of raised intracranial pressure. However, they may also present with behavioral problems and focal seizures, particularly if arising within a temporal lobe. Magnetic resonance imaging is the imaging modality of choice and in many cases will be diagnostic or at least give valuable clues as to which other investigation should be undertaken. Cerebral computed tomography (CT) should be avoided wherever possible because it does not reveal the same range of abnormalities as MRI and subjects the infant to considerable radiation (3). There are certain circumstances in which imaging may not be mandatory (e.g., a patient with neonatal hypoxic–ischemic encephalopathy and previous [diagnostic] imaging, who subsequently develops epilepsy will probably not require repeat MRI unless epilepsy surgery is being considered as a treatment option). Where the initial imaging is reported to be normal in the early infantile period, repeat scanning may be indicated at a later date if seizures persist. Subtle developmental lesions may be difficult to visualize on MRI until myelination is more complete at the age of 18–24 months. It is important to understand that high-resolution (at least 3.0 Tesla) MRI may be the most relevant repeat scanning technique and this will necessitate referral to a tertiary epilepsy centre.

Chromosomal disorders

In the absence of a readily recognizable cause for the infant's epilepsy, chromosome analysis should be a mandatory investigation. Chromosomal anomalies are quite frequent when epilepsy is accompanied by other major congenital abnormalities such as congenital heart disease or cranio-facial abnormalities. However, even in the absence of other somatic abnormalities (including dysmorphic facial features), current high-resolution chromosome analysis may identify small deletions or duplications.

Some chromosome abnormalities have a very high rate of epilepsy as part of their phenotype:

- The majority of patients with Wolf–Hirschhorn syndrome caused by deletions in the short arm of chromosome 4 have early-onset epilepsy along with other congenital abnormalities and characteristic facial features (Greek helmet-shaped face).
- Approximately 8–10% of children with trisomy 21 will develop West syndrome (infantile spasms).
- Ring chromosome 20 is commonly associated with drug resistant seizures, although the onset is rarely in early infancy but usually in early childhood.

More detailed genetic investigations may be warranted for infants with unclassified epilepsy and a learning disability (mental retardation), with or without any soft dysmorphic features. Telomere studies and Multiple Ligation-dependent Probe Amplification (MLPA) are relatively new techniques which can detect microscopic deletions in specific regions. These investigations should always be taken in conjunction and following discussion with clinical geneticists.

Metabolic disorders with epilepsy in infancy

Although many children with inborn errors of metabolism may develop epilepsy, most do not present primarily with epileptic seizures, or manifest seizures in isolation. Inborn errors of metabolism are extremely important to consider and diagnose because many are potentially treatable. Potential clues to an underlying metabolic etiology include:

- a family history of neonatal or infantile death
- parental consanguinity
- micro- or macrocephaly
- developmental impairment
- failure to thrive or short stature
- hepatomegaly

- other organ dysfunction
- uncommon seizure types, and specifically myoclonic or tonic seizures.

Mitochondrial and peroxisomal disorders are becoming increasingly recognized as a cause of infantile epilepsy.

Potentially treatable causes of early infantile epilepsy which may significantly improve developmental and cognitive functioning include:

- **biotinidase deficiency** (4). This diagnosis is suggested by the combination of alopecia, eczema and neurological problems including seizures. However, many infants may show only some of these features. Urine organic acid analysis and measurement of the biotinidase level will establish the diagnosis and prompt but lifelong treatment with biotin supplementation may allow a relatively good outcome
- **disorders of glucose transportation** (5) into the central nervous system. This is diagnosed by finding inappropriately low levels of glucose in the cerebro-spinal fluid (CSF) (neuro-glycopenia) or a low fasting CSF: blood glucose ratio (< 0.35). The phenotype of this relatively recently described disorder is expanding rapidly (including patients with what appears to be drug resistant absence epilepsy or patients without epilepsy) and is potentially treatable by the ketogenic diet
- **pyridoxine-dependency** (6). This rare disorder **must** always be considered in any infant with drug resistant epilepsy and usually without an identified etiology. Approximately two-thirds of patients present with neonatal seizures but pyridoxine-dependency can also present at any time in the first 18–24 months of life with developmental impairments and epilepsy. The usual presentation after the neonatal period is with very frequent myoclonic seizures or infantile spasms; the EEG may show a burst-suppression or atypical hypsarrhythmic pattern.

Most common specific epilepsy syndromes in early infancy

The most common – and also potentially the most difficult to treat – include the following:

- West syndrome
- severe myoclonic epilepsy of infancy (Dravet syndrome)
- migrating partial seizures in infancy
- benign infantile convulsions.

West syndrome

This is probably the most common recognizable epilepsy syndrome which occurs in early infancy with an incidence of approximately 0.31/1,000 live births. The earliest description in modern medical literature was provided by Dr William West. Dr West wrote a heartbreaking letter to the editor of the *Lancet* asking for advice about his own son. In this letter he exquisitely describes the seizure semiology, the clustering pattern of the seizures and the associated developmental stagnation/regression. In the 1950s, various authors, notably Gibbs and Gibbs, described the associated EEG abnormality, hypsarrhythmia.

West syndrome (WS) is commonly defined on the basis of infantile spasms and a hypsarrhythmic EEG; developmental impairment or regression, if not already present at the time of the diagnosis of WS, nearly always evolves and will be obvious before the end of the first year of life. The onset is usually within the first year of life with a peak around six to eight months of age. Rarely, WS can present after the first year of life with infantile spasms in isolation and without a hypsarrhythmic EEG or developmental regression or, even less commonly, with a hypsarrhythmic EEG but no spasms. These situations usually occur in the context of a child with severe preceding neurological disability and the symptoms or signs may be overlooked by parents, care-givers or health professionals.

Presenting symptoms: The most common presenting symptom is with the pathognomic seizure type – the infantile spasm. Infantile spasms have been called various names including jack-knife seizures, and salaam attacks. The seizures have an insidious onset, gradually increasing in frequency before presentation. They may initially be mistaken for infantile colic or an exaggerated startle response even by healthcare professionals. Spasms have various appearances. In a time-synchronized video/polygraphic monitoring study, Kellaway *et al.* described different types of spasms including flexor, extensor, asymmetrical and spasms associated with motor arrest (7). The majority exhibited a mixture of different types of spasms. In practice, differentiating between different types of spasms does not usually provide clues to the underlying etiology with the exception that persistently asymmetrical spasms may be associated with a unilateral hemispheric abnormality. The 'classical' description of a spasm that accounts for 50–70% of cases is with sudden flexion of the head, neck and trunk with abduction of the arms followed by a few seconds of sustained tonic contraction. The infant recovers but may be upset for 10–30 seconds and then another spasm occurs. This may be repeated with three to four to over a hundred spasms occurring in a cluster. Spasms can be much more subtle, sometimes involving isolated muscle groups such as the abdominals or ocular muscles or the neck. These spasms are obviously much harder to recognize and may require simultaneous video–EEG monitoring to be well defined. There are often other clinical manifestations associated with the spasms. The child is upset and cries after a spasm or may be relatively unresponsive. The clustering of infantile spasms is typically within a few minutes after waking or, slightly less frequently, as the infant is falling asleep. Spasms rarely occur during sleep.

Some degree of developmental regression usually accompanies the onset of the spasms, although more commonly it develops after the onset of the spasms. The developmental regression can manifest itself in a number of ways. In cryptogenic infantile spasms the infant may have been developing normally before the onset of spasms and then becomes progressively lethargic, disinterested in their surroundings and eventually appears to be blind. This may occasionally result in the infant being referred to ophthalmology services with visual loss, particularly if the spasms are subtle. In a child with severe pre-existing neurological disorders such as severe neonatal hypoxic–ischemic encephalopathy or following severe meningitis in the newborn period, the developmental regression may be more subtle or even absent. Parents may only notice an improvement in behavior or development once the spasms and accompanying hypsarrhythmia are treated.

Unless the underlying etiology is obvious (e.g., neonatal hypoxic–ischemic encephalopathy or Down syndrome), a search for an underlying cause must always be undertaken. Approximately 80% of children will have an identifiable cause and should therefore be classified as symptomatic West syndrome. With improvements in brain imaging and in medical genetics, the list of underlying etiologies has grown with, consequently, a gradually shrinking proportion of those with 'cryptogenic' causes – those in whom no cause is found. Initial investigation should, as always, begin with the history and examination. The pregnancy and peri-natal history is important as is the early development prior to spasm onset. Family history may also important; familial cases of infantile spasms are uncommon but a history of intellectual disability, especially in males, can be an important clue. Examination may reveal skin stigmata of a neuro-cutaneous syndrome such as tuberous sclerosis, the most common single cause of infantile spasms. Examination of the parents is important because tuberous sclerosis is inherited as an autosomal dominant disorder with variable expression. Ophthalmological examination may provide further information such as the retinal 'punched out' lacunae of Aicardi syndrome. The most important single investigation is the MRI brain scan, which may identify many of the other structural abnormalities which can cause WS, including neuronal migration disorders, and may provide clues to an underlying neuro-metabolic (specifically a mitochondrial) disorder. Basic genetic investigation should include good-quality, high-resolution chromosome analysis to identify disorders including inverted duplication of the pericentric region of chromosome 15. Further investigations can then be planned focusing on neuro-metabolic investigation and more detailed genetic analysis. Even following extensive investigations there remain a proportion of patients without an identifiable cause, the group with 'cryptogenic' or 'idiopathic' WS.

Diagnosis: The diagnosis of WS is usually obvious. Parental description of the events with their characteristic clustering is usually enough to point the clinician towards the diagnosis. Further information on developmental regression may be available. All patients with WS must have at least a standard EEG recording to demonstrate hypsarrhythmia, the electrical hallmark of infantile spasms. This is also useful to assess the infant's response to treatment.

Hypsarrhythmia is present in approximately 70–80% of patients with infantile spasms. Difficulties arise when the history is highly suggestive of infantile spasms but the initial EEG is normal or, if abnormal, non-hypsarrhythmic. An EEG should then be obtained during sleep or, ideally, the infant should undergo simultaneous video–EEG recording to capture events.

A number of different disorders, broadly divided into epileptic and non-epileptic, may mimic infantile spasms including normal sleep myoclonus, normal physiological Moro reflex, shuddering attacks or startle disease. Because of the brief, transient nature of infantile spasms they may be confused with other epileptic seizures, most commonly myoclonic seizures. Benign myoclonic epilepsy may present at a similar age but is less common than WS. The very brief tonic phase of infantile spasms and their tendency to occur in clusters and soon after waking are characteristic and are not seen in infants with myoclonic seizures.

Severe myoclonic epilepsy of infancy (Dravet syndrome and other SCN1A-related epileptic encephalopathies)

Dravet syndrome is a relatively rare (although probably under-recognized) but important epilepsy syndrome of early infancy. It was first described by Charlotte Dravet, a French neurologist, in 1982 (8, 9). The original term was 'severe myoclonic epilepsy of infancy' (SMEI), and the two names have been used interchangeably over the years. However, the eponym Dravet syndrome is generally considered the preferred term because myoclonic seizures are not usually the predominant seizure type and may not even occur in every patient. There is – and continues to be – much interest in this syndrome with the discovery that the majority of patients with Dravet syndrome have an identifiable mutation in the sodium ion channel gene SCN1A (9).

Clinical presentation: Children with classical Dravet syndrome present in the first year of life with prolonged seizures, usually with febrile illnesses or in association with an intercurrent illness. Typically the child presents with an episode of febrile status epilepticus (generalized or commonly hemiclonic) at between four and eight months of age. The hemiclonic seizures often seem to alternate in side from seizure to seizure. The clinician should become suspicious of the syndrome by the fact that the seizures are not simply recurrent complex febrile seizures and by the frequency of the events, the prolonged nature of the seizures, the fact that the body temperature may not be very elevated (38°C–38.5°C) and the precipitating effect of environmental heat such as hot water baths. In between seizures the child is well and appears to be making 'normal' developmental progress.

During the second and third year of life the convulsive seizures persist and become more frequent but of shorter duration. At this time other and more fulminant seizure types develop and include myoclonic, partial (focal) and atypical absences. Myoclonic seizures can be dramatic, sometimes resulting in falls (so-called massive myoclonias). Atypical absences are associated with loss of awareness, head nods, falls, or sometimes with myoclonic seizures. The atypical absences may become prolonged, leading to periods of non-convulsive status epilepticus. One of the hallmarks of this epilepsy syndrome is the developmental stagnation/regression which usually begins in the second or third year of life and mirrors the evolution of multiple seizure types and periods of non-convulsive status epilepticus. Children with Dravet syndrome may also become ataxic and develop mild pyramidal tract signs, usually in the middle to end of the first decade of life.

Diagnosis: The diagnosis of Dravet syndrome is based on the evolution of the epilepsy phenotype. Frequent febrile or afebrile convulsions during the first year of life and particularly alternating hemiconvulsions should alert the clinician to the possibility of Dravet syndrome. The age at diagnosis seems to be decreasing (Dr SM Zuberi – personal communication), which almost certainly reflects an increasing awareness of the disorder and, consequently, early genetic investigation.

The EEG is usually normal in the first 12 to 18 months, despite the high frequency of prolonged seizures (8). Generalized and focal EEG abnormalities begin to be noted in the second year of life but are not specific for the syndrome. Approximately 40% of those with Dravet syndrome demonstrate a photoparoxysmal response (PPR), sometimes as early as the first year of life, and this early onset PPR can suggest the diagnosis. EEGs undertaken in the third year of life onwards demonstrate increasingly slow-wave activity. Neuro-imaging with either CT or MRI is usually normal – even when the syndrome has become well established.

Approximately 80% of patients with classical Dravet syndrome have a mutation in a gene which codes for a neuronal sodium channel, SCN1A. The majority of patients with Dravet syndrome have de novo mutations in this gene, although there are a few reports of familial cases, presumably as a result of gonadal mosaicism in one of the parents. Mutations in other ion channel genes SCN2B and GABA-B have also been found in a small proportion of patients with Dravet syndrome. Gene-testing for SCN1A mutations is now readily available (through the British Pediatric Neurology Association [BPNA] website). It is important to understand that SCN1A mutations are associated with many other types of epilepsy, which means that an SCN1A mutation confirms but does not diagnose Dravet syndrome (10). Finding the cause for such a devastating epilepsy syndrome can be extremely helpful to parents/carers and enables clinicians to make an early diagnosis without having to undertake numerous, and potentially invasive, investigations.

Migrating partial seizures in infancy (MPSI)

This recently delineated syndrome appears to be very rare. Migrating partial seizures in infancy is one of the most severe epileptic encephalopathies or catastrophic epilepsies seen at any age in childhood (11, 12). Seizures respond poorly if at all to anticonvulsants and the clinical progression is usually one of relentless developmental regression. The underlying cause has yet to be identified and the diagnosis is based on the description of the seizures and supporting EEG features.

Clinical presentation: Seizures begin in the first year of life, usually before three to four months and even in the first week of life. Infants appear normal at birth and family history and clinical examination is unremarkable. The seizures are partial (focal) but involve different body areas and sides from one seizure to the next. Autonomic features are very common during the seizures with flushing, tachycardia, pallor and epiphora (eye-watering). The onset is usually explosive with frequent seizures which occur in clusters. Seizure-frequency may vary from less than ten to over a hundred per day, and usually every day. Progressive microcephaly, presumably caused by failure of normal brain growth, occurs in the first year of life. Infants with

MPSI fail to make any meaningful developmental progress after the onset of the seizures and any skills acquired before the onset of epilepsy are usually lost.

The inter-ictal EEG is usually normal. Ictally, seizures are seen to arise independently from various regions of the brain, sometimes with one seizure terminating in one region as another starts in another region, hence the term 'migrating partial seizures'; this frequently occurs during a single EEG recording. This characteristic finding, in an otherwise normal infant, should raise the possibility of this diagnosis, although a careful search for other etiologies should still be made, including structural and metabolic disorders (specifically, mitochondrial disorders and pyridoxine-dependency).

Benign epilepsy syndromes of early infancy

Benign infantile seizures

This is a relatively rare epilepsy syndrome of early infancy. In common with benign neonatal convulsions, there are familial (usually autosomal dominant) and non-familial forms (13). The syndrome was first described by Japanese authors in the 1960s and further delineated by Watanabe in the early 1980s.

Clinical presentation: Familial and non-familial benign infantile convulsions present in a similar fashion, although the familial group on average present a little earlier in life (six months versus nine months). A previously normal child will have a sudden onset of brief seizures, usually occurring in a cluster over a 24-hour period with good recovery in between seizures. Seizures may recur over the next few days to weeks but will eventually stop spontaneously, usually towards the end of the first year of life. The seizures are focal, sometimes with secondary generalization. In a seizure, there will be a sudden behavioral arrest followed by head and eye deviation to the side, generalized hypertonia, perioral cyanosis and sometimes oral automatisms. Rhythmical clonic jerks may be seen, sometimes bilaterally.

Diagnosis: In non-familial cases, the diagnosis of benign infantile convulsions should always be one of exclusion. Given the high frequency of acute symptomatic and symptomatic focal epilepsies in this age group a careful search should be made for any precipitating factors. Investigations should include basic biochemistry (blood electrolytes, glucose, calcium, liver function etc.), neuro-imaging (MRI) and a search for infection including cerebrospinal fluid analysis. Paired fasting blood and CSF glucose measurements will usually exclude glucose transporter (GLUT-1) deficiency. The diagnosis of non-familial infantile convulsions is most secure in hindsight! In familial cases, the seizures are transmitted in an autosomal dominant manner. Sometimes the diagnosis is easily made because the child is part of a large pedigree with many family members being affected over several generations. A grandmother most often provides the most accurate family history. Further investigations are not required if the history is obvious and examination findings are normal.

The inter-ictal EEG is almost always normal. Occasionally there may be mild slowing of the background but this is often caused by the effects of medication rather than the underlying epilepsy. Ictal records are difficult to obtain as seizures have usually resolved by the time any prolonged EEG recordings are available.

There are a number of similar bur rarer 'benign' focal epilepsies of early infancy. Benign familial neonatal–infantile seizures occupy a borderline between benign familial neonatal seizures and benign infantile seizures. The clinical features of this syndrome are similar to benign familial infantile seizures except that the age of onset is much earlier, typically between three days and three months. Mutations in the SCN2A gene, a voltage-gated sodium channel, are found in a number of large families with benign familial neonatal–infantile seizures, which provide further evidence of the importance of ion channelopathies in the underlying pathogenesis of many of the epilepsy syndromes (13).

Benign myoclonic epilepsy in infancy

This is a rare disorder with an onset between six months and three years but usually around 12 months of age (14). The only seizure type is myoclonus. Affected children are otherwise well with normal neuro-development. The myoclonic seizures are brief and usually obvious, affecting the head, trunk and upper limbs; less commonly they may be more subtle with head nods and eyelid flickering. The seizures rarely cause the child to fall. They behave and play normally as soon as the seizure has stopped. The inter-ictal EEG is often normal but the ictal EEG usually shows a generalized polyspike and slow-wave discharge associated with the myoclonic seizure. The epilepsy resolves over the next few years. Recently, some investigators have suggested that with longer-term follow-up, some children do demonstrate significant cognitive problems.

Early treatment of infantile epilepsies

General considerations

As with epilepsy at any age, management must begin with the correct diagnosis. The clinician must always ask the question 'Is this epilepsy?' not only at the time of diagnosis but during follow-up visits. The differential diagnosis of epilepsy at this age may be complex and the many mimickers of epilepsy in infancy can cause diagnostic difficulties. A 'trial of antiepileptic medication' is never justified when there is doubt about the diagnosis.

Once the diagnosis of both the epilepsy and seizure type (and ideally, epilepsy syndrome) is secure the next step is to decide on the most appropriate medication with the goal of seizure freedom without side effects. Because many of the early-onset epilepsies are severe and difficult to treat, this goal may prove impossible to achieve. To monitor the effect of treatment, the commonly used modality is parental reports on seizure frequency and severity. This is typically undertaken in out-patients, although in some of the more severe early-onset epilepsy syndromes, children may remain in hospital for considerable periods of time as a result of massive seizure burden and its consequences. In some situations it may be necessary to repeat an EEG to monitor treatment. This is particularly important in West syndrome, because it is hypothesized that hypsarrhythmia rather than the spasms is the more important factor in determining developmental and cognitive outcome, as well as the underlying cause. This is because hypsarrhythmia can be considered as non-convulsive status epilepticus. In addition, more prolonged EEG recordings may identify subtle spasms and other seizures that are not recognized by either the child's parents or clinicians.

The concept of treatment-effectiveness should also include freedom from side effects. As with assessing effectiveness, the occurrence of side effects will be based on parental reports; it is therefore important to make parents/carers aware of the more likely and certainly important side effects of any medication. Subtle changes in behavior and levels of alertness can be difficult to assess in this age group.

Serum anticonvulsant level monitoring is controversial and the practice is largely dependent on geographical location and the philosophy of local tertiary units. With the exception of phenytoin and phenobarbitone, both of which have a very narrow therapeutic window, routine monitoring of levels is not widespread in either the United Kingdom or in Canada. In certain situations, a random blood level may assist the assessment of possible drug toxicity or suspected major non-adherence. In addition, the protein-binding of a drug, individual sensitivity to side effects, a wide 'therapeutic range' and correct timing of blood samples make serum concentration monitoring difficult.

The antiepileptic medication should be chosen that is most appropriate for the seizure type (15). For example, carbamazepine or levetiracetam would be reasonable choices for the majority of infants with focal seizures, but in a child with a congenital hemiplegia who develops infantile spasms (presumably secondary to a seizure focus in the affected hemisphere), carbamazepine would be inappropriate; it would be unlikely to stop the spasms and may exacerbate them. Care should be taken with the use of sodium valproate in infancy because of the risk of fatal hepatotoxicity in this age group. The rate has been reported to be as high as 1 in 500 infants under the age of two/three years although this is likely an overestimate (16). It should be noted the majority of cases of fatal hepatotoxicity have occurred in infants with early-onset and severe epilepsy (which typically includes myoclonic seizures) and severe developmental delay. It is possible that many of these patients had an underlying metabolic condition, including a urea cycle or mitochondrial disorder, and specifically Alpers' disease (17).

Finally, the chosen drug should be available in an infant-friendly preparation. This usually means a liquid preparation but increasing numbers of anticonvulsant medications are available in other forms including powders which can be dissolved (e.g., vigabatrin) or granules (e.g., topiramate) which can be sprinkled on food or in liquids for ease of administration.

Specific treatment of individual syndromes

West syndrome

The treatment of West syndrome (WS) is controversial and is guided in part by clinicians' experience and training, local protocols and geographical availability of medications. The first-line treatment of West syndrome is nearly always either hormonal treatment (ACTH [tetracosactide], prednisolone, hydrocortisone) or vigabatrin. Randomized trials have established that both treatments can be effective but it remains somewhat unclear which treatment is more effective and particularly on long-term developmental outcome (18). Most randomized comparative trials report that hormonal treatment has a slightly greater chance of suppressing the spasms than vigabatrin, but with higher rates of side effects. A number of studies have shown that WS caused by tuberous sclerosis complex responds better to vigabatrin than steroids (18). Ideally, future randomized trials should focus on specific etiologies.

The balance between seizure-suppression and side effects has lead many clinicians to start treatment with vigabatrin and move promptly to hormonal treatment if there is no response after one or two weeks. Even though this approach seems intuitively correct, it remains unclear if very prompt (within one or two weeks) suppression of seizures improves the long-term developmental outcome in West syndrome.

Response to therapy should be monitored not only by spasm frequency but by resolution of the hypsarrhythmic pattern on the EEG. Some authors suggest that a positive response to treatment should only be considered after a prolonged period of EEG monitoring, including during slow-wave sleep, to confirm the complete resolution of hypsarrhythmia and absence of spasms, some of which may be subtle and unrecognized by parents/carers. This approach is obviously costly. In addition the very rare situation may arise where the spasms cease but the hypsarrhythmia persists. The dilemma is then to decide to 'treat the EEG or the patient'; this is complex and should obviously only be addressed by specialists from a tertiary centre.

Hormonal treatment: This involves treatment with either oral steroids (prednisolone, betamethasone, hydrocortisone) or injected corticotrophin stimulating agents (usually ACTH or the synthetic analog, tetracosactide). There is no clear evidence as to which is the more effective, although many clinicians sense that ACTH/tetracosactide is more effective than prednisolone or hydrocortisone (18). Hormonal treatment with ACTH is given by daily or occasionally twice daily intramuscular injections, which are painful and may be associated with more side effects. A suggested treatment regime for ACTH and prednisolone is shown in Table 2.1. Spasms, when they respond to hormonal therapies, often respond very quickly, sometimes within the first 24–48 hours and an 'all or nothing' response is often seen – as it may be with vigabatrin after 72 to 120 hours (five days). Current practice would indicate that steroid treatment should be given for at least two weeks before considering it ineffective.

The main side effects include irritability, weight gain, alterations in glucose and electrolyte homeostasis, hypertension and, rarely, death caused by septicemia.

Table 2.1 Suggested treatment regimens with ACTH, prednisolone and vigabatrin

Drug	Starting dose	Suggested regime	Important side effects
ACTH (tetracosactide)	500 μg intramuscularly alternate days	Continue for two weeks then reduce dose by 50% for two weeks then by further 25% for two weeks then stop	Irritability almost inevitable. Hypertension, hyperglycemia, immune suppression leading to overwhelming sepsis and death (rare)
Prednisolone	2–4 mg/kg once daily	Continue for two weeks. If no response discontinue. If complete response wean steroid dose over six-week period	As above although tendency to be less pronounced compared with ACTH
Vigabatrin	25 mg/kg twice daily	Increase every six doses by approx. 12.5 mg/kg/dose to a maximum 75 mg/kg twice daily	Irritability, lethargy, hypotonia, GI upset. Visual field loss which may be permanent (rare in this age group)

Because of the risks of immunosuppression parents must be warned about the risk of infection and specifically any exposure to chicken pox. Many units issue 'steroid-alert' cards for parents and carers.

Vigabatrin: Vigabatrin is many clinicians' first choice in the treatment of WS. In general it is far better tolerated than hormonal therapy, even allowing for the high doses and rapid escalation used in this condition. In contrast with steroid therapy, administration of vigabatrin does not require careful monitoring of blood pressure, electrolyte and blood glucose. It may, if effective, be continued for longer periods of time than steroids and is thought to be associated with a lower relapse rate. A treatment regime is suggested in Table 2.1.

The primary if only concern with vigabatrin is a serious and permanent deleterious effect on visual fields. This results in (usually) asymptomatic and bitemporal visual loss which appears not to resolve with discontinuation of the drug (19, 20); however, this reported irreversibility has been predominantly reported in adult-treated populations. The incidence in adults is considered to be approximately 40%; the incidence in children is difficult to ascertain but is considered to be approximately 25%. Visual fields can only be reliably assessed in children with a developmental age of at least nine years. In addition many patients with WS will have severe developmental disability, making formal assessment very difficult at any age. The visual field deficit has resulted in some clinicians avoiding the use of vigabatrin.

Other therapies: Between 30–60% of children with West syndrome will not respond to either vigabatrin or hormonal therapy. Evidence for other therapies is limited and mainly limited to case series (18). Benzodiazepines (mainly nitrazepam but alternatively, clonazepam or clobazam) have been used for many years and it is our experience that nitrazepam (and occasionally sodium valproate) are particularly useful when the cause of WS is secondary to peri-natal acquired lesions. They may be used either as monotherapy or in combination with vigabatrin or sodium valproate. However, these combinations may cause some drowsiness.

Pyridoxine (vitamin B6) may rarely be remarkably effective in West syndrome, although this is nearly always restricted to those infants where the underlying cause is pyridoxine dependency. Other anticonvulsants may be of some use in West syndrome although the data are very limited. These include sodium valproate (usually in high doses of > 60 mg/kg/day), topiramate and zonisamide. These drugs can be introduced and increased relatively rapidly and may suppress spasms as well as abolish hypsarrhythmia.

Dravet syndrome (SMEI)

Treatment of Dravet syndrome is difficult because of the multiple seizure types and their drug resistance and should only be undertaken in conjunction with a specialist in pediatric epilepsy. Stiripentol in combination with valproic acid and clobazam is the only drug regime that has been subjected to a randomized trial in Dravet syndrome and appears to significantly reduce seizure frequency and particularly the generalized tonic-clonic seizures (21). Stiripentol is not readily accessible in many countries and is relatively expensive. Because of the multiple seizure types in Dravet syndrome and its broad spectrum of action, sodium valproate is generally the drug of first choice (15). A benzodiazepine, usually clobazam or clonazepam, is often used in conjunction with valproate. Another and often effective combination is valproate with either topiramate or zonisamide. Stiripentol (along with valproic acid and clobazam) should be considered sooner rather than later, although it may be associated with significant sedation or irritability; this is probably related to the fact that three drugs are being used simultaneously, an approach that should be avoided wherever possible. Low-dose phenobarbital may also be effective, either as monotherapy or in combination with either sodium valproate or zonisamide. The ketogenic diet and short courses (four to six weeks) of prednisolone may also be effective in some children. Finally, it is important to emphasize that lamotrigine, carbamazepine and phenytoin may dramatically exacerbate the seizures in Dravet syndrome and should generally be avoided (22).

Benign infantile epilepsies

Many children with benign infantile epilepsies will not require regular treatment with an antiepileptic drug. Seizures often occur in clusters lasting 24 hours with complete recovery between them. In this situation, the use of intermittent benzodiazepines (termed 'rescue medication') administered buccally (midazolam) or rectally (diazepam) can be useful. For example, parents can be instructed to give a benzodiazepine if the infant has three seizures within an hour. The apparent rarity of these syndromes means that there is no information as to which drug should be prescribed for those infants who require prophylaxis for frequent seizures; low-dose carbamazepine or sodium valproate could be used, obviously depending on the seizure type or epilepsy syndrome.

Middle treatment of infantile epilepsies

General considerations

The treatment of epilepsy at any age does not begin and end with the diagnostic process. Depending on the type of epilepsy syndrome, follow-up of infants with epilepsy must be a long-term process, ending only if the epilepsy enters spontaneous remission; if the epilepsy remains active, follow-up must continue through transition and into adult life.

For many of the symptomatic epilepsies presenting in early infancy, seizure management will only represent a small part of the health needs of the child. Infants who had experienced moderate to severe neonatal hypoxic–ischemic encephalopathy will require access to a multi-disciplinary neuro-developmental team in order to maximize developmental potential, monitor feeding and facilitate access to education.

Access to nursery placements, both mainstream and special, should be available and where appropriate nursery staff should be trained in the administration of any rescue medication. Children with Dravet syndrome often present particular challenges because of the severity and duration of some seizures and their very ready provocation by even mild intercurrent illness. A clear and explicit protocol for treatment of convulsive status epilepticus is required for whoever cares for the child – whether their parents, baby-sitter/child-minder or nursery school.

Information on compliance or adherence with antiepileptic medication should be sought at clinic visits. This is obviously entirely in the hands of the infant's carers. There may be specific difficulties in getting the infant to take preparations of antiepileptic medication; alternative preparations should be used if administration becomes difficult. It is also important to enquire about other concomitant medications that the child may be receiving because this may cause clinically relevant drug interactions; this is crucial in children with severe neuro-disability who are often taking large numbers of concomitant medications.

Infants undergo vaccinations or immunizations as part of their routine healthcare. It is important that these be administered and, wherever possible, at the appropriate times. Having epilepsy, irrespective of the epilepsy syndrome or cause, and receiving antiepileptic medication (of any type, other than corticosteroids) do not constitute contraindications for the administration of these vaccines.

Co-morbidities in infantile epilepsies

Learning and development

Because of the often severe nature of underlying symptomatic etiologies and often frequent seizures in infantile epilepsies, early developmental attainments and learning may be impaired or previously acquired skills lost. This may also apply to those infants in whom no cause for the epilepsy has been identified. This is well illustrated by infants with drug resistant cryptogenic/presumed symptomatic West syndrome. An infant with apparently normal early development begins to lose previously attained skills around the onset of spasms. Conversely, a rapid and sustained clinical and EEG response to treatment in WS can lead to a recovery of lost skills, particularly visual behavior and social interaction. Nevertheless, despite this recovery, most infants with even cryptogenic WS are left with significant intellectual disability. The precise relationship between the seizures, EEG changes and developmental impairment is as yet unknown and remains an active area of research. A study of infants with WS caused by trisomy 21 showed that those diagnosed (and therefore treated) after eight weeks showed a poorer response in terms of spasm suppression and had a poorer developmental outcome and showed more autistic features; this was not entirely related to persistence of spasms in the group of children diagnosed after eight weeks (23). This suggests that both early and effective treatment for West syndrome is critical. Clearly, these data need to be confirmed in other groups of infants with WS caused by specific etiologies.

Family adjustment

Epilepsy that occurs at any age can be very distressing and may cause significant and often intolerable stress on the family, including older siblings. This is particularly significant in those families where the child is an infant (with their 'whole life ahead of them') and the seizures are frequent and often prolonged, resulting in frequent hospitalizations. These children also experience school difficulties not only because of the effect of frequent seizures and persistently 'epileptic' activity on the EEG, but also through disrupted school attendance. It is obviously very important that parents be given honest and realistic advice about their child's epilepsy as well as the support and access to medical services that they will frequently require. Epilepsy nurse specialists are extremely valuable in these situations, establishing a clear link between the hospital-based services and the child's home and school.

What to do if the first drug fails?

The failure of a first antiepileptic drug (AED) to control seizures should lead to a careful reappraisal of the child's problem including:
- have they been receiving the antiepileptic medication on a regular and consistent basis?
- does the child really have epilepsy?
- if 'yes,' has the correct seizure type and epilepsy syndrome been diagnosed?
- has an underlying cause been considered and actively sought?

It is always important to ask about the development of any new paroxysmal events or seizure types: myoclonic and some focal seizures can be subtle, easily overlooked or dismissed by parents/carers. Sometimes the correct syndrome will only become apparent over time, and this may be months rather than weeks. For example, children with Dravet syndrome present with febrile tonic-clonic seizures in the first year of life and the myoclonic and absence seizure only subsequently present in the second or third year of life.

A review of the seizure type and syndrome may also include repeating investigations and specifically the EEG. Prolonged video–EEG recordings are useful if any doubts remain about the nature of paroxysmal events. The possibility that the patient may have one of the early-onset neuro-degenerative disorders should also be considered, even if there were no clues to this diagnosis at the onset. Failure to achieve developmental milestones or even loss of previously acquired milestones, changing or new neurological symptoms and signs, abnormal head growth (acquired micro- or macrocephaly) or even subtle behavioral changes can all be important clues to a possible underlying neuro-degenerative disorder. Prominent myoclonic seizures in particular are often associated with the neuro-degenerative disorders and specifically a metabolic disorder. The most commonly encountered metabolic disorders at this age will be late infantile neuronal ceroid lipofuscinosis ('Batten's disease') and progressive neuronal degeneration of childhood with or without liver disease (Alpers' disease).

Other than poor seizure control as determined by the natural history of the epilepsy syndrome, the next most common reason for failure of a first medication is an unacceptable side effect. Many side effects in infancy are predictable and can be reduced or avoided by slow-dose titration. However, rapid changes in hepatic and renal elimination of drugs can give rise to rapid changes in plasma concentration as the infant grows; this is particularly illustrated by phenytoin, a difficult drug to titrate at the best of times, although fortunately this drug is only rarely used in the treatment of the infantile epilepsies.

Once the decision to change medication has been made the first decision is whether to directly substitute medication and maintain monotherapy, or whether to use combination therapy. In general, sequential monotherapy should be the principle, and combination therapy reserved until there have been at least two attempts at monotherapy. If treatment with multiple antiepileptic drugs is required (as occasionally in WS and very commonly in Dravet syndrome and migrating partial seizures in infancy), the number should be kept to a minimum, and ideally no more than two used simultaneously. Three drugs should be used only very rarely; first, because there are no convincing data that three are more effective than two, and second because of the risk of adverse side effects, including on the infant's development and behavior.

Syndrome-specific therapy

Middle treatment of WS will depend on the response to initial treatment. If complete seizure control is achieved with resolution of the hypsarrhythmic EEG pattern, vigabatrin is usually continued for approximately four, or at most, six months before being withdrawn. When spasms stop with hormone treatment, usually the hormone treatment is gradually withdrawn over one to three months; there is a higher risk and rate of relapse if withdrawal is over one month. If spasms return, then a second course of hormone treatment is often undertaken and if that fails then vigabatrin or other more conventional medications such as sodium valproate or nitrazepam will be prescribed, possibly determined by the underlying etiology.

Alternative treatments for epilepsy in infancy

Epilepsy surgery

Epilepsy surgery, with techniques initially developed in adult practice and subsequently modified for the pediatric population, is the only current therapy that can result in a 'cure' for refractory epilepsy. It is important to both appreciate and emphasize that surgery can, and should, be performed whenever this is appropriate. This includes in infants and young children because years of frequent and drug resistant epilepsy may result in irreversible cognitive (educational) and behavioral consequences which could potentially be prevented by early and curative surgery.
   There are two main types of operation:
- Resective surgery – the objective is to remove the epileptogenic zone or lesion responsible for the seizures (24).
- Palliative surgery – the objective is to reduce the frequency or severity of seizures, sometimes by targeting specific seizure types, and specifically 'drop attacks' (tonic or atonic seizures). The two main types of palliative procedure are corpus callosotomy (25) and vagal nerve stimulator implantation (26).
Consideration of epilepsy surgery is reserved for patients with medically refractory epilepsy. There is no unanimous definition of 'medically refractory epilepsy' but pragmatically it is generally defined as a failure to achieve 12 months' seizure freedom with a minimum of two or possibly three appropriately prescribed antiepileptic medications. There are however a number of situations

where epilepsy surgery should be considered early in the course of the disease. These include:

- Infants with primary brain tumors who present with epileptic seizures
- Sturge–Weber syndrome. This is a good example of a disorder in which the natural history of the disease (refractory epilepsy, progressive hemiplegia, progressive cognitive impairment) can be altered by early resective surgery – in this case hemispherectomy or hemispherotomy (the latter term refers to disconnection rather than removal of the abnormal hemisphere).

A perhaps more common epilepsy syndrome which may be amenable to surgery is West syndrome and where there is an obvious focal lesion including focal cortical dysplasia, a porencephalic cyst (secondary to a congenital or peri-natally acquired stroke) or an epileptogenic tuber in tuberous sclerosis. Reported seizure freedom rates in selected groups of patients are as high as 65% and most of these patients have already failed with many antiepileptic drug treatments. It is tempting to consider that early targeted surgical treatment may improve neuro-developmental and cognitive outcome in a proportion of children with an infantile epilepsy.

The role of vagal nerve stimulation (VNS) in the treatment of all the epilepsies, and particularly the epilepsy syndromes of infancy, remains uncertain. Although technically more difficult in infants, VNS can and has been undertaken in migrating partial seizures of infancy, Dravet syndrome and West syndrome (26).

Ketogenic diet

The ketogenic diet, with appropriate instigation, close dietetic monitoring and follow-up, is a viable option for infants with medically refractory epilepsy who are unable to undergo epilepsy surgery (27). There are currently three variants:

- Classical (largely food-based).
- Medium chain triglyceride (MCT; largely liquid-based). This is the preferred variant for infants with feeding gastrostomy tubes *in situ*.
- Modified Atkins (the most 'relaxed' and least restricting of the three variants).

The traditional ('classical') ketogenic diet is carefully calculated to provide a certain ratio (grams of fat : grams of protein and carbohydrate) which usually ranges 3–4 : 1. The other two variants (median chain triglyceride [MCT] and modified Atkins) are generally more palatable and therefore better tolerated – particularly in older children (28, 29). The MCT variant is usually the more appropriate one to use in infants and young children, who are fed through a feeding gastrostomy tube.

There are two rare disorders, pyruvate dehydrogenase complex deficiency and glucose transporter (GLUT-1) deficiency syndrome, for which the treatment of choice is the ketogenic diet. The seizures and movement disorders in these conditions often show a dramatic response. The ketogenic diet is being increasingly used earlier in the course of the epilepsy when initial medications fail in many infants with other metabolic disorders or epilepsy syndromes. Evidence suggests that the infant brain is better than the adult brain in utilizing ketone bodies as an alternative energy substrate. It is also clear that the diet is better tolerated in infants and young children than in teenagers and adults.

The diet must be adhered to tightly and this can be difficult or impossible for the infants and their families. Assuming it is closely adhered to, a period of at least four to eight weeks will be adequate to determine if it has been effective and whether it should be continued (a good response) or withdrawn (no response or a poor response).

In terms of efficacy, most of the published data on the use of the ketogenic diet in infancy is in the more severe epilepsy syndromes and particularly West and Dravet syndromes. Overall, it seems that approximately one-third of these infants will have a good response to the diet. One non-randomized, retrospective study compared ACTH and the diet as the initial treatment of infantile spasms and found no statistical difference in efficacy or time to spasm freedom (30), although ACTH was close to showing a superior effect (p = 0.06). Predictably, there was a lower incidence of side effects in infants treated with the diet. However, it must be recognized that the diet is both an abnormal and complex diet and infants will require vitamin and mineral supplements and close clinical, biochemical and hematological monitoring. Nevertheless, the diet does merit consideration early in the course of the infantile epilepsies, particularly in the more severe epilepsy syndromes, including migrating partial seizures in infancy. It can only be initiated, and closely monitored by a tertiary epilepsy centre.

Later treatment of infantile epilepsies

Prognosis of epilepsy presenting in infancy

As might be expected, the prognosis of the more severe epilepsy syndromes of early infancy is generally poor in terms of the seizure outcome and, perhaps more importantly, the cognitive (particularly communication) and behavioral outcome. The outcome of the benign syndromes is generally good although the risk of later specific cognitive problems is probably still slightly greater than that of the general population.

West syndrome

Despite improvements in recognition of WS and the availability of newer treatments, published data from various sources (particularly Finland) suggest that the long-term outcome of infants with WS has not changed markedly over the past thirty years (28). The prognosis depends primarily on the underlying etiology. There is a small group of patients with normal early development prior to the onset of spasms, classical hypsarrhythmia, normal investigations including normal neuro-imaging and an excellent and sustained response to initial treatment that will have a normal or near normal cognitive outcome. This group, which constitutes between 5 and 10% of all infants with WS, is sometimes referred to as idiopathic WS, often because there is a strong family history of epilepsy, but not usually WS. Obviously, it may not be that easy to identify this group at initial presentation. In general however, the prognosis of

West syndrome is usually very poor. In a large series from Finland, 65% of all patients had severe learning disability (intelligence quotient or developmental quotient less than 50), 76% still had epilepsy at the age of three and over 10% had a symptomatic generalized epilepsy (31). These figures are very similar to reports in the 1960s and 70s. The main factor which predicted a poor outcome was having a symptomatic etiology (32). Finally, there remains a slightly increased mortality rate which also has not changed significantly over the years; by 3 years of age 13% of the patients had died compared with 11% in the historical control group.

Dravet syndrome

Unfortunately, the long-term prognosis of Dravet syndrome is very poor. Children are usually developmentally normal prior to the onset of seizures. This is always followed by a regression in development which then plateaus at around five or six years of age. Overall intelligence in older school children is typically severely affected (10). Conflicting evidence suggests that either language and communication, or visuo-spatial skills are predominantly affected. Behavioral difficulties are also frequent as manifest by hyperactivity, impulsivity and autistic traits. Seizures usually persist although they may become less problematic as the patient gets older with the atypical absences and myoclonic seizures becoming less frequent and the tonic-clonic seizures being of shorter duration. Motor impairment, specifically acquired ataxia, is also seen in older children with Dravet syndrome and may be related to the dysfunction of sodium channels in the cerebellum or the seizures themselves, or a combination of factors.

Long-term studies of children with Dravet syndrome have suggested that the frequency of convulsive seizures (more than five a month) is associated with a worse cognitive outcome. It is therefore tempting to speculate that better initial control of seizures may improve cognitive outcome in these children. It remains to be seen if the use of more aggressive therapies including stiripentol or the ketogenic diet could alter the natural history of this devastating epilepsy syndrome. Finally, there is an increased mortality in Dravet syndrome as a result of convulsive status epilepticus, accidents including drowning and, possibly more importantly, sudden unexpected death in epilepsy (SUDEP). Approximately one in seven children with Dravet syndrome die before adolescence.

Migrating partial seizures in infancy

Although this is a relatively recently reported syndrome (and more long-term data are clearly required), the vast majority of infants show a very poor or poor outcome. This encompasses both seizure frequency and developmental functioning. In addition, a number of infants have died under five years of age, occasionally earlier.

Outcome of the benign epilepsy syndromes of infancy

The outcome of benign infantile convulsions, both familial and non-familial, is excellent with normal development and cognitive function. Seizures do not recur, even in the patients who require treatment during infancy. There is no generally agreed consensus on how long these patients require treatment; it seems reasonable to treat for approximately six to twelve months and then withdraw medication.

Benign myoclonic epilepsy of infancy is also reported to have a good outcome in terms of seizure control with the majority responding well to sodium valproate and spontaneous remission of seizures over a period of time. However, the cognitive outcome may not be as good. A recent literature review indicated that approximately one-third of patients had some degree of learning disability ranging from mild specific learning disability to more severe global cognitive impairments (13).

REFERENCES

1. Camfield CS, Camfield PR, Gordon K, Wirrell E, Dooley JM. Incidence of epilepsy in childhood and adolescence: a population-based study in Nova Scotia from 1977 to 1985. *Epilepsia* 1996; **37**: 19–23.
2. Sheth RD, Bodensteiner JB. Effective utilization of home-video recordings for the evaluation of paroxysmal events in pediatrics. *Clin Pediatr* 1994; **33**: 578–82.
3. Berrington de González A, Mahesh M, Kim KP, *et al.* Projected cancer risks from computed tomographic scans performed in the United States in 2007. *Arch Intern Med* 2009; **169**: 2071–7.
4. Wolf B. Clinical issues and frequent questions about biotinidase deficiency. *Mol Genet Metab* 2010; **100**: 6–13.
5. Leen WG, Klepper J, Verbeek MM, *et al.* Glucose transporter-1 deficiency syndrome: the expanding clinical and genetic spectrum of a treatable disorder. *Brain* 2010; **133**: 655–70.
6. Basura GJ, Hagland SP, Wiltse AM, Gospe SM Jr. Clinical features and the management of pyridoxine-dependent and pyridoxine-responsive seizures: review of 63 North American cases submitted to a patient registry. *Eur J Pediatr* 2009; **168**: 697–704.
7. Kellaway P, Hrachovy RA, Frost JD Jr, Zion T. Precise characterization and quantification of infantile spasms. *Ann Neurol* 1979; **6**: 214–18.
8. Dravet C, Bureau M, Oguni H, Fukuyama Y, Cokar O. Severe myoclonic epilepsy in infancy: Dravet syndrome. *Adv Neurol* 2005; **95**: 71–102.
9. Arzimanoglu A. Dravet syndrome: from electroclinical characteristics to molecular biology. *Epilepsia* 2009; **50**(Suppl 8): 3–9.
10. Scheffer IE, Zhang YH, Jansen FE, Dibbens L. Dravet syndrome or genetic (generalized) epilepsy with febrile seizures plus? *Brain Dev* 2009; **31**: 394–400.
11. Coppola G, Plouin P, Chiron C, Robain O, Dulac O. Migrating partial seizures in infancy: a malignant disorder with developmental arrest. *Epilepsia* 1995; **36**: 1017–24.
12. Caraballo RH, Fontana E, Darra F, *et al.* Migrating focal seizures in infancy: analysis of the electroclinical patterns in 17 patients. *J Child Neurol* 2008; **23**: 497–506.
13. Specchio N, Vigevano F. The spectrum of benign infantile seizures. *Epilepsy Res* 2006; **70**: (Suppl 1): S156–67.
14. Dravet C, Bureau M. Benign myoclonic epilepsy in infancy. *Adv Neurol* 2005; **95**: 127–37.
15. Wheless JW, Clarke DF, Arzimanoglou A, Carpenter D. Treatment of pediatric epilepsy: European expert opinion. *Epileptic Disord* 2007; **9**: 353–412.
16. Bryant AE 3rd, Dreifuss FE. Valproic acid hepatic fatalities. III. US experience since 1986. *Neurology* 1996; **46**: 465–9.

17. Bicknese AR, May W, Hickey WF, Dodson WE. Early childhood hepatocerebral degeneration misdiagnosed as valproate hepatotoxicity. *Ann Neurol* 1992; **32**: 767–75.
18. Hancock EC, Osborne JP, Edwards SW. Treatment of infantile spasms. *Cochrane Database Syst Rev* 2008 Oct 8; **4**: CD001770.
19. Kälviäinen R, Nousiainen I. Visual field defects with vigabatrin: epidemiology and therapeutic implications. *CNS Drugs* 2001; **15**: 217–30.
20. Wild JM, Chiron C, Ahn H, *et al.* Visual field loss in patients with refractory partial epilepsy treated with vigabatrin: final results from an open-label, observational, multi-centre study. *CNS Drugs* 2009; **23**: 965–82.
21. Chiron C, Marchand MC, Tran A, *et al.* Stiripentol in severe myoclonic epilepsy in infancy: a randomised placebo-controlled syndrome dedicated trial. STICLO study group. *Lancet* 2000; **356**: 1638–42.
22. Guerrini R, Dravet C, Genton P, *et al.* Lamotrigine and seizure aggravation in severe myoclonic epilepsy. *Epilepsia* 1998; **39**: 508–12.
23. Eisermann MM, DeLaRailliere A, Dellatolas G, *et al.* Infantile spasms in Down syndrome – effects of delayed anticonvulsive treatment. *Epilepsy Res* 2003; **55**: 21–7.
24. Saneto RP, Wyllie E. Epilepsy surgery in infancy. *Semin Pediatr Neurol* 2000; **7**: 187–93.
25. Yang TF, Wong TT, Kwan SY, *et al.* Quality of life and life satisfaction in families after a child has undergone corpus callosomy. *Epilepsia* 1996; **37**: 76–80.
26. Zamponi N, Rychlicki F, Corpaci L, Cesaroni E, Trignani R. Vagus nerve stimulation (VNS) is effective in treating catastrophic epilepsy in very young children. *Neurosurg Rev* 2008; **31**: 291–7.
27. Kossoff EH, Rho JM. Ketogenic diets: evidence for short- and long-term efficacy. *Neurotherapeutics* 2009; **6**: 406–14.
28. Kossoff EH, *et al.* A modified Atkins diet is effective for the treatment of intractable pediatric epilepsy. *Epilepsia* 2006; **47**: 421–4.
29. Pfeifer HH, Thiele EA. Low glycaemic-index treatment: a liberalized ketogenic diet for treatment of intractable epilepsy. *Neurology* 2005; **65**: 1810–2.
30. Kossoff EH, Hedderick EF, Turner Z, Freeman JM. A case–control evaluation of the ketogenic diet versus ACTH for new-onset infantile spasms. *Epilepsia* 2008; **49**: 1504–9.
31. Riikonen R. Long-term outcome of patients with West syndrome. *Brain Dev* 2001; **23**: 683–7.
32. Riikonen RS. Favourable prognostic factors with infantile spasms. *Eur J Paediatr Neurol* 2010; **14**: 13–18.

3

Epilepsy beginning in middle childhood

Elaine Wirrell and John H. Livingston

The history

The diagnosis of epilepsy is critical to its management; the first question that must always be asked, and answered as fully and as comprehensively as possible, is whether the cause of the child's paroxysmal episodes are epileptic in nature (1).

In the majority of cases the diagnosis is made from the history alone. An invaluable aid is being able to review a video recording of an episode. This is increasingly available at the first consultation with video cameras on most mobile phones. This also requires skill and episodes may still be difficult to diagnose. Watching the video with the parents and/or child is important and useful and it is sometimes a humbling experience to recognize how difficult it is to describe the events that parents and observers witness, and particularly the range of movement disorders.

If the clinician is unable to recount the attack from beginning to end in their 'mind's-eye', they are likely to be uncertain about the nature of the paroxysmal episode. For example, a generalized tonic-clonic seizure may be the end point of many different focal seizure types. It is the most dramatic and frightening aspect of the seizure and may be all that parents can remember or focus on. Unless specific questions are asked about the onset and offset of the seizure, or about other clinical features, the correct diagnosis may be missed. It is also important not to forget to take a history from the child even if very young. For example, a description of a fuzzy feeling inside the mouth before a nocturnal tonic-clonic seizure is highly suggestive of a rolandic seizure, or a young child may be able to draw a visual hallucination or describe a feeling of being scared, which might suggest an occipital or temporal lobe origin respectively.

Childhood Epilepsy: Management from Diagnosis to Remission, ed. Richard Appleton and Peter Camfield. Published by Cambridge University Press. © Cambridge University Press 2011.

When the diagnosis is uncertain or seizures continue in spite of treatment it is always worth reviewing and checking the history again from the beginning. This takes time and it is important to allow for this when planning outpatient consultations.

Acute presentation of seizures

While most epileptic seizures are acute events, the occurrence of a seizure in the context of an acute illness must always raise the question as to whether the seizure is symptomatic of an acute CNS insult, i.e., that it is an 'acute symptomatic seizure.' The most important aspect in this situation is to diagnose correctly and give the appropriate treatment for the acute disorder.

As with any epileptic seizure, misdiagnosis is common and this can have serious and sometimes fatal consequences (2). The most important misdiagnosis to be aware of is mistaking tonic extensor spasms for epileptic seizures. Epileptic tonic seizures do not usually occur as a single seizure type and usually occur as part of a mixed severe epilepsy such as Lennox–Gastaut syndrome or in a child with a severe underlying brain abnormality.

A previously well child presenting acutely with repetitive tonic seizures, and particularly in association with a depressed conscious level, has acutely raised intracranial pressure and is about to 'cone' until proven otherwise.

This child must not be given a benzodiazepine before appropriate investigation and management for raised intracranial pressure and the prevention of 'coning' (herniation).

The management of acute seizures will be different according to whether the seizure is continuing when the child arrives in hospital or not. The management of status epilepticus is considered elsewhere. Guidelines for acute seizure management generally refer to generalized tonic-clonic seizures. If it is uncertain whether the seizure is epileptic or not then a further specialist opinion should be obtained or appropriate investigations undertaken, or both.

The most common cause for an acute epileptic seizure in infancy is a febrile seizure. Guidelines for the investigation of simple febrile seizures have been published (3). Acute seizures in a febrile child require further investigation when there are other neurological signs or symptoms and particularly focal signs, when the conscious level has not returned to normal within 30 minutes of the seizure ending (4), repeated (serial) short seizures or status epilepticus. In any of the above situations and where there is a strong suspicion of meningitis or encephalitis, antibiotics and antivirals should be commenced pending the results of further investigations.

Debate continues as to when a lumbar puncture should and should not be undertaken in a febrile child. The following provides a useful guideline:

Lumbar puncture following a seizure in a febrile child
- *Indications*
  - complex febrile seizure in a child < 12 months
  - suspected CNS infection
  - unexplained status epilepticus
- *Contraindications*
  - depressed conscious level 30 mins after seizure cessation
  - new focal neurological signs
  - signs of raised intracranial pressure, especially tonic seizures/extensor posturing
  - intracranial lesion on CT causing a mass effect or ventriculomegaly
  - active coagulopathy or thrombocytopenia (< 10,000)

Investigations are directed at identifying the cause of the seizure and particularly in those who may need urgent medical or surgical treatment (Table 3.1).

Table 3.1 Investigations for a child presenting acutely with epileptic seizures

Afebrile:
- blood glucose
- blood calcium and magnesium
- blood urea and electrolytes
- CT scan

If febrile the child may also require:*
- blood and urine cultures
- consider lumbar puncture
- other investigations should be dictated by the clinical picture

If diagnosis unclear, save urine and blood for possible future investigations

*(depending on the specific clinical situation)

Acute imaging will be necessary in many, but not all children. Febrile seizures rarely require neuro-imaging. Other acute presentations where imaging may not be necessary include: a simple metabolic derangement such as hypoglycemia or hypocalcemia, and a firm diagnosis of a familial infantile epilepsy syndrome in a neurologically normal child. Imaging will generally be required in the following circumstances: when the etiology is unknown, there are focal neurological signs, there is alteration of conscious level or failure to return to normal consciousness within 30 minutes of a short seizure (4), status epilepticus or suspected non-accidental injury. Computerised tomography (CT) is the imaging modality of choice in the emergency situation and where there is a strong suspicion of meningitis or encephalitis, intracranial hemorrhage or hydrocephalus. Magnetic resonance imaging (MRI) with specific sequences may be useful if the child is considered to have experienced a stroke.

The presentation and differential diagnosis of epilepsies starting in childhood

An epilepsy or an epileptic seizure is usually suspected because a child has had a paroxysmal event. The parents may or may not suspect that the event was epileptic in nature. It is important to think of the ways in which seizures may first come to the notice of parents or other witnesses and to consider the differential diagnoses of each of these categories. This is particularly important when the child comes with a medical label already attached.

The most common ways in which epileptic seizures may present
- staring/blank spells
- falls
- falls with 'convulsions'
- abnormal movements
- events during sleep
- abnormal behaviors

Staring, blank spells or 'absences'

Episodes of apparent unresponsiveness with or without staring are extremely common in young children and a common reason for referral to a pediatrician. The majority of these episodes are non-epileptic and represent 'day dreaming' or thought immersion. Important features in the history are the context, frequency, timing and duration of the episode as well as nature of onset and offset and the presence of associated features – such as eyelid fluttering/flickering, blinking, eye movements, automatisms (lip-smacking, chewing, hand-fidgeting) and color change. Most non-epileptic staring episodes occur infrequently and not every day and tend to last much longer than epileptic attacks. They are also rarely completely stereotyped with exactly the same pattern of behavior occurring in each attack. Unlike absence seizures, non-epileptic staring spells can be interrupted with stimulation such as tickling the child or blowing on their face.

Differential diagnosis of non-epileptic blank spells/staring episodes
- thought immersion – engrossed in a task (e.g., watching television, on a computer)
- day dreaming
- self-gratification
- pre-syncopal (e.g., supraventricular tachycardia)
- nausea
- hyperventilation

Epileptic blank spells can be a manifestation of a generalized seizure (an absence) or a focal seizure (a simple or complex partial or focal seizure).

Typical absence seizures occur in a number of different idiopathic generalized epilepsy syndromes, the most common being childhood absence epilepsy which is discussed later; these absences usually occur many times a day and last from 10 to 30 seconds.

Focal (previously termed complex partial) seizures are commonly preceded by some specific symptoms, or non-specific symptoms that are often described as an 'aura' – which is in fact the onset of the seizure (although younger children may not be able to describe precisely what they feel). They occur far less frequently than absence seizures, are of longer duration (even lasting many minutes) and are accompanied by focal features including unilateral automatisms, head or eye deviation or dystonic posturing, and are often followed by post-ictal confusion or tiredness, or both. Children will often sleep following a focal seizure, even if it lasts only a minute or so.

An accurate history will usually be able to differentiate non-epileptic from epileptic blank spells. However, it may be more difficult to do this accurately in a child who is already neurologically abnormal or who also has other epileptic seizures.

Falls

Children who fall 'for no apparent reason' are often referred for evaluation of possible epilepsy. The differential diagnosis of 'falls' is large. Epileptic 'drop attacks' are usually fairly dramatic events and often result in injuries. The history usually allows the diagnosis to be made. Epileptic drop attacks may be caused by atonic, tonic or myoclonic seizures and usually co-exist with other seizure types which should be specifically asked about and specifically absence, myoclonic or clonic seizures. The seizures do not only happen while the child is ambulant and may be as subtle as a brief head nod or jerk seen during meal times or while playing games or watching television.

Differential diagnosis of non-epileptic falls
- ataxia (episodic or chronic)
- weakness
  - peripheral neuropathy
  - periodic paralyses
  - myasthenia
- cataplexy
- syncope
- myoclonus
- startle disease (hyperekplexia)
- paroxysmal movement disorders

Fall with abnormal movements or convulsions

The archetypal epileptic seizure in the minds of both lay people and many health professionals is the generalized tonic-clonic seizure (or 'grand mal' as it is still often referred to). If a child falls and develops abnormal movements it is almost invariable that a diagnosis of an epileptic seizure is made. The most common misdiagnosis is labeling syncope as an epileptic seizure because stiffening or brief and even repeated jerking of limbs frequently occurs during a syncopal attack (5). This may occur whatever the mechanism for the syncope, which causes transient cerebral hypoxia – with the most common causes being vasovagal, reflex anoxic seizure or cardiogenic (as in an arrhythmia). In general the more profound the impairment of cerebral perfusion and degree of cerebral hypoxia, the more likely are abnormal movements to occur. The most common movements are tonic or dystonic stiffening followed by a few myoclonic or clonic jerks and the movements may be symmetric or asymmetric. If clonic jerking persists for more than a few seconds this is not consistent with syncope and is more likely to be an epileptic seizure. A rare occurrence is when a syncopal episode triggers a true epileptic seizure; this is called an anoxic epileptic seizure (6).

The occurrence of a tonic or 'convulsive' seizure during or following fairly vigorous exercise should suggest the possibility of cardiogenic syncope and must be investigated further.

Distinguishing features between syncope and generalized tonic-clonic seizures

	Syncope	Generalized tonic-clonic seizure
Aware of onset	Yes: light-headedness and gradual visual loss common	No: unless it is a secondary generalized tonic-clonic seizure which has followed an aura
Sudden collapse	Sometimes but may have time to sit down or seek support	Yes
Muscle tone on collapsing	Limp initially; may then become stiff	Stiffening of arms and or legs, clenching teeth
Jerking (myoclonic or clonic)	Four or five jerks after collapse	Continuous jerking arms and legs, fast at first then slowing
Usual duration of jerking	Few seconds	30 seconds to 2 minutes
Eye-rolling (tonic upgaze)	Sometimes with stiffening	Yes
Cyanosis	Sometimes	Often
Post-episode tiredness	Yes	Yes
Incontinence	Sometimes	Frequently (not always)

In an older child or young teenager the other relatively common cause of a fall followed by 'convulsive' movements is a so-called non-epileptic attack, which is most appropriately termed a 'psychogenic non-epileptic seizure.' These attacks are very uncommon in children under seven years of age.

Abnormal movements

The differential diagnosis of paroxysmal movement abnormalities is large and a comprehensive discussion is beyond the scope of this chapter. An epileptic basis to such movements is commonly considered and misdiagnosis is common. A good history provided from an eye-witness and supported by video documentation will usually enable the correct diagnosis. The diagnosis is particularly challenging in a neurologically abnormal child or when the child has definite epileptic seizures; in both situations clinicians may be tempted to assume that any paroxysmal disorder must represent an epileptic seizure with consequent misdiagnosis. If these attacks are prolonged, they may (rarely) be misdiagnosed as 'status epilepticus', leading to inappropriate management with potentially serious iatrogenic complications. Video recordings may again be helpful, if not diagnostic, but occasionally EEG monitoring may be particularly helpful. Some movements are highly likely to be epileptic (e.g., focal clonic movements), others are sometimes epileptic (e.g., myoclonus), while others are rarely epileptic (e.g., chorea, athetosis or ballismus).

Differential diagnosis of paroxysmal movements
- an epileptic seizure
- paroxysmal dyskinesias
- tics
- myoclonus
- episodic ataxia
- startle responses
- reflux-induced dystonia
- shuddering spells or attacks
- extensor spasms caused by tonsillar herniation
- self-gratification phenomena
- stereotypies/mannerisms (particularly common in children with moderate or severe learning difficulties)
- non-epileptic attack disorder (specifically psychogenic, non-epileptic seizures)

Events during sleep

Epileptic seizures commonly occur during sleep or during the night. There are many other non-epileptic sleep-related phenomena (which collectively are often termed 'parasomnias') that are relatively commonly misdiagnosed as epilepsy. Nocturnal frontal lobe seizures may be difficult to distinguish from night terrors; useful differentiating features seen in nocturnal frontal lobe seizures include:

- the episodes are brief (10–60 seconds in duration, only rarely longer)
- the episodes (seizures) occur several times per night
- the episodes may occur through the night (night terrors tend to occur about 90 minutes after falling asleep)
- the episodes usually involve dystonic posturing or stereotyped hyperkinetic movements
- the same episodes may also occur when awake.

In the rare syndrome autosomal dominant nocturnal frontal lobe epilepsy (ADNFLE), one of the parents may give a history of sleep disturbance themselves that has not been recognized as epileptic or has been labeled as 'paroxysmal nocturnal dsytonia'). Video recordings of the child's episodes may prove diagnostic, but may be confirmed by overnight video–EEG recording and polysomnography if the diagnosis remains uncertain. However, seizures arising from the mesial frontal lobe may show no electrical change on a surface (scalp) EEG even when recorded during the seizure. Finally, it is important to recognize that there are sleep disorders that remain poorly characterized; this again emphasizes the importance of keeping an open mind and never rushing to diagnose epilepsy when there is doubt or uncertainty.

Events that occur during sleep
- epileptic seizures[*]
  - frontal
  - temporal
  - occipital
  - idiopathic focal
(*any of these seizures could end in a generalized tonic-clonic seizure)
- night terrors
- nightmares
- sleep myoclonus (specifically benign neonatal, but at all ages)
- head-banging and other sleep–wake transition disorders

Abnormal behavior

Another common reason for referral for suspected epilepsy is the child who is having episodic abnormal behavior, especially rages or tantrums. In an otherwise normal child it is exceptionally rare for paroxysmal rage or aggression to be the only manifestation (and presenting feature) of an epilepsy. Children with episodes of sudden, unexplained and often extreme rage or anger that last many minutes and which may be followed by exhaustion and no recall of the episodes may have the episodic dyscontrol syndrome, also termed intermittent explosive disorder. Other behavior changes, and specifically confusion, behavioral arrest, staring and automatisms are common features of an epileptic seizure, including in a prolonged generalized absence seizure (typical or atypical), temporal lobe seizure or other focal seizure. These attacks are usually stereotyped and are not usually situation-dependent. Paroxysmal fear or fright, which can be sudden and alarming for observers, is relatively common in childhood complex partial (focal) seizures and particularly in those arising from the temporal lobe. Other features often occur which support an epileptic basis, including eye and/or head deviation and dystonic posturing of a limb (typically an arm). Post-ictal tiredness and sleep are also characteristic of a focal seizure.

Bizarre motor behaviors may be a feature of an epileptic seizure but these are usually stereotyped, such as walking round in a circle or sitting or jumping up and down repeatedly.

Children experiencing hallucinations (whether epileptic or non-epileptic), will often exhibit bizarre behaviours, which may be difficult to understand if the child is young or unable to give a history.

Non-convulsive status epilepticus primarily presents with behavioral changes. These are usually regressive in nature rather than a positively directed behavior and are most often manifest by:
- deterioration in speech or even speech arrest (mutism)
- loss of concentration
- ataxia
- drooling
- sudden paucity of movement in children who are usually hyperactive (e.g., as in Angelman and Rett syndromes).

There are often associated motor features including jerking or atonic seizures. Non-convulsive status epilepticus in childhood almost always develops in a child who has a pre-existing diagnosis of epilepsy and usually a more severe epilepsy such as Lennox–Gastaut syndrome, myoclonic–astatic epilepsy (also known as Doose syndrome, and severe myoclonic epilepsy of infancy (also known as Dravet syndrome). Non-convulsive status epilepticus arising for the first time in a child without epilepsy is very rare but has been described usually as part of an idiopathic generalized epilepsy syndrome and particularly if treated with antiepileptic drugs such as carbamazepine, phenytoin and vigabatrin.

Narcolepsy is characterized by excessive daytime sleepiness, cataplexy, sleep paralysis and hypnagogic hallucinations. Cataplexy is often misdiagnosed as a 'drop' or atonic seizure; in cataplexy the episodes of sudden falls or 'drops' (like a puppet's strings being cut) are always provoked – usually by laughter or a sudden shock and the child remains on the floor, fully conscious but unable to move. The diagnosis in young children is often delayed and behavior problems may be prominent.

Episodic abnormal behaviors
- epileptic seizures
  - temporal lobe
  - frontal and occipital
  - other unclassified focal
  - prolonged absence
  - non-convulsive status epilepticus
- temper tantrums
- episodic dyscontrol syndrome (also called intermittent explosive disorder)
- conduct disorder
- anxiety disorder
- psychosis
- self-gratification phenomena
- excessive daytime sleepiness
  - cataplexy and narcolepsy

Regression with or without epileptic seizures

Loss of previously acquired skills (motor or cognitive) may have an epileptic basis. When this occurs, it is usually in a child who already has a pre-existing diagnosis of epilepsy, and specifically epileptic spasms, frequent atypical absences or tonic-clonic seizures. Rarely, regression may be the only manifestation of the epilepsy and it is only when an EEG is undertaken that it is recognized that there may be an epileptic basis to it, with the demonstration of frequent or very frequent sharp wave, spike and wave or polyspike and wave activity. This is particularly the case with the syndromes associated with continuous spike and wave of slow-sleep (CSWSS), including electrical status epilepticus of slow wave sleep (ESESS) or the Landau–Kleffner syndrome. A sleeping EEG should always be undertaken in a child with regression in whom a waking EEG shows frequent sharp wave or spike and slow-wave activity. The diagnosis of CSWSS and ESESS will obviously be missed if a sleeping EEG is not performed. This is important because more aggressive treatment, not necessarily of the child's seizures, but more importantly the markedly abnormal EEG, may reverse some of the child's loss of skills and allow developmental and cognitive progress.

In a child with epilepsy, regression may be caused by the seizures, the treatment or by an underlying progressive etiology.

Regression with epileptic seizures
- neuro-degenerative disease
  - genetic, e.g., neuronal ceroid lipofuscinoses (NCLs), mitochondrial cytopathies and Huntington's disease
  - acquired including subacute sclerosing panencephalitis (SSPE) and systemic lupus

- antiepileptic drug toxicity (rare)
- the epilepsy itself
  - epileptic encephalopathies (e.g., Ohtahara, West and Dravet syndromes; CSWSS)
  - very frequent seizures
- psychiatric co-morbidity
  - depression
  - psychosis
  - drug toxicity

Specific epilepsies that present in childhood

The classification of the epilepsies is yet again undergoing revision (7) with a view to encompassing new knowledge as well as abandoning old concepts which may no longer be valid; however, any new classification is likely to be temporary and change with further advances in molecular genetics. The concept of the epilepsy syndrome is likely to continue to be useful as a way to describe groupings of clinical, electrical or other features that characteristically occur together.

In the next section the common epilepsy syndromes that present in childhood will be considered. Many children have an epilepsy that cannot be easily fitted into existing syndrome definitions. The clinician has to steer a path between the need to give meaningful information to patients and make pragmatic decisions about therapy and the need to keep an open mind about revising the initial diagnosis in the light of new information and clinical features as and when these become available.

Childhood absence epilepsy (CAE)

CAE is one of the most common epilepsies presenting in childhood and is one of the idiopathic generalized epilepsies. It is genetically determined and is likely to involve several or multiple susceptibility genes as well as other genetic and even environmental factors.

The peak age of onset is five to seven years. Absences starting before two years or after ten years should suggest an alternate diagnosis. Females are affected approximately three times more commonly than males.

The hallmark seizure is the typical absence characterized by abrupt onset and termination, severe impairment of awareness and interruption of ongoing activity. The eyes usually open and stare, sometimes with mild blinking or flickering/fluttering of the eyelids or periorbital muscles. Automatisms are common, including lip-smacking or chewing. Duration is usually between 5 and 20 seconds. Recovery is rapid with no post-ictal tiredness or sleep.

Typically absences occur very frequently, from 10 to over 100 a day, every day. If they are infrequent a different diagnosis should be considered.

Absences are readily triggered by hyperventilation and this is a procedure that should be undertaken in the outpatient clinic. Hyperventilation should be performed for at least three minutes.

The EEG has a normal background and demonstrates 3 cycles/second generalized spike and wave with abrupt onset and offset. The discharges usually slow towards the end of the seizure.

Other seizure types may occur in CAE although authors differ in their opinion as to whether this is acceptable, in terms of a 'pure' diagnosis of CAE. Using very strict criteria (8), no other seizure types occur in CAE. However, using slightly less strict criteria, generalized tonic-clonic seizures (GTCS) are reported to occur in 16 to 45% of patients.

The prognosis is generally favorable and approximately 60–65% of absences will spontaneously remit before 12 years of age. Some patients go on to develop GTCS which are usually easily controlled.

Typical absence seizures may occur in other idiopathic epilepsies of childhood including myoclonic–astatic epilepsy (MAE) and epilepsy with myoclonic absences. Juvenile absence epilepsy (JAE) may occasionally present in younger children and absences may be the presenting seizure type of juvenile myoclonic epilepsy (JME); the absences in JAE and JME are often of longer duration. Other syndromes in which absences may occur include: eyelid myoclonia with absences and perioral myoclonia with absences. Childhood absence epilepsy may be one of the syndromes that occur in the genetic epilepsy syndrome 'GEFS Plus' or 'GEFS+' (generalized epilepsy with febrile seizures plus) (9).

Rarely, typical absences may arise from a focal source in the medial frontal lobe or temporal lobe. If absences are drug resistant, or are associated with focal features (e.g., head deviation consistently to one side), MRI should be performed.

Benign focal epilepsies of childhood (also known as idiopathic focal epilepsies)

These epilepsies are common in childhood, representing up to 25% of epilepsies that occur in children under 16 years of age.

Benign epilepsy with centro-temporal spikes (BECTS) (also known as benign rolandic epilepsy of childhood [BREC] or benign childhood epilepsy with centro-temporal spikes [BCECTS]) accounts for two-thirds of patients with benign focal epilepsy syndromes.

The peak age of onset is between five to eight (range two to14) years. Seizures are infrequent with only one seizure in 10%, two to six seizures in 70% and only 20% have frequent seizures.

The classic seizure is a clonic seizure involving one side of the face, often preceded by numbness or tingling (sometimes described by the child as 'fizzing') of the tongue, inside of the cheek or lips. The child is unable to speak normally (dysarthria) but contact is preserved. The seizures are brief, lasting one or two minutes, and may spread to the arm and rarely the leg, or evolve into a secondary GTCS.

Seizures occur only during sleep in 70% of children. Far less commonly they occur only during wakefulness.

The EEG typically shows high-amplitude biphasic sharp waves in the centro-temporal (rolandic) area which become much more frequent during drowsiness and sleep. In around 30% of patients they are only present during sleep.

The prognosis for seizure remission is excellent with remission by the age of 15 or 16 and usually within two to four years of onset. Generally the cognitive outcome is excellent. However, some behavioral and neuro-psychological difficulties, particularly in communication skills, have been reported both during the active period of seizures and on follow-up. The frequency and interpretation of this continues to be the subject of debate (10).

Panayiotopoulos syndrome is a benign focal epilepsy syndrome that is often misdiagnosed in view of the fact that the predominant symptomatology is autonomic (11, 12). It is reported to represent at least one-third of the benign focal epilepsy syndromes, although this remains under debate.

The typical seizure begins with pallor, nausea and sometimes vomiting. There may be hypersalivation and other autonomic features including flushing, cyanosis or sweating. The child may become unresponsive and floppy. Eye deviation is common and the seizure may evolve into a hemiclonic seizure involving face or limbs and ultimately may generalize. However, the frequency of these features varies considerably in affected children. Seizures are prolonged in around half of cases and may last 30 minutes or longer. Recovery is usually rapid.

These seizures are often misdiagnosed as encephalitis, metabolic disease or migraine and sometimes a child is admitted to intensive care and undergoes extensive investigations. This is understandable and probably appropriate if it represents the child's first seizure.

As with BECTS seizure frequency is reported to be generally low, with a single seizure in 25%, two to five in 50% and rarely very frequent seizures.

The EEG reveals multifocal spikes, often with an occipital preponderance. The background is usually normal.

The prognosis is considered to be excellent with complete remission of seizures within one to two years of onset. Some children may develop rolandic seizures or, less commonly, occipital seizures.

Idiopathic childhood occipital epilepsy of Gastaut (also known as late-onset childhood occipital epilepsy or benign partial epilepsy with occipital paroxysms [BEOP]) is a less common idiopathic focal epilepsy syndrome with a mean age of onset of eight years.

The seizures primarily manifest with elementary visual hallucinations and are often frequent, short and occur during wakefulness.

Most characteristically the hallucinations comprise small multicolored circular patterns in the periphery of the visual field, moving horizontally during the course of a seizure (12). Other features include eye and head deviation, ictal blindness, headache, vomiting, and less commonly focal or generalized clonic seizures.

The EEG shows occipital paroxysms which often appear when fixation on an object is eliminated.

An MRI is indicated as symptomatic occipital epilepsies may have identical clinical features.

The prognosis is less certain than for the other idiopathic focal epilepsies. Approximately 60% will remit within four years, however some continue to have seizures long term.

Epileptic encephalopathies

Epileptic encephalopathy
This is defined as: 'An epilepsy that has an adverse effect on cerebral function (encephalopathy) resulting in cognitive and/or neurological impairment.' Implicit in the term is the concept that the encephalopathy is the consequence of the epilepsy, resulting from very frequent clinical seizures, continuous or semi-continuous paroxysmal EEG activity (spike and wave), or both.

Epileptic encephalopathies presenting in childhood
- myoclonic–astatic epilepsy (MAE)
- Lennox–Gastaut syndrome
- Dravet syndrome (seizure onset is in infancy but epileptic encephalopathy develops later)
- continuous spike-wave of slow-sleep (CSWSS)
- Rassmussen syndrome
- severe symptomatic epilepsies – including those caused by neuro-degenerative and/or metabolic disorders

---

Epilepsy with myoclonic–astatic seizures (also known as Doose syndrome) is characterized by the occurrence of myoclonic–astatic seizures together with other seizure types. The 'hallmark' seizure involves a typically symmetrical myoclonic seizure followed by sudden loss of muscle tone (atonic seizure). This results in the child falling or losing posture: the 'astatic' seizure.

Myoclonic–astatic epilepsy (possibly to be termed in the future classification, myoclonic-atonic epilepsy [MAE]) is currently regarded as an idiopathic generalized epilepsy in which genetic factors are important. It may occur in families with GEFS+ which may occur in association with mutations in the *SCN1A*, *SCN1B* or *GABRG2* genes (13). The peak age of onset is between two and four years and there is a slight male preponderance.

The typical presentation is a child who repeatedly falls because of drop attacks, often hurting themselves. If the seizures are less severe there may be simply head nods or a brief slump forward without a complete fall. The seizures may evolve gradually or there may be a more explosive onset with rapid escalation in seizure frequency. Other seizure types may precede, coincide or follow the myoclonic–astatic seizures. The most common seizure types are: generalized tonic-clonic seizures, absence seizures, atonic seizures and febrile convulsions. Tonic seizures may occur, although some would consider this seizure type as precluding this syndrome. The presence of tonic seizures would suggest more that the child has the Lennox–Gastaut syndrome. Myoclonic–astatic seizures may occur in other epilepsies, and particularly severe symptomatic epilepsies. Lennox–Gastaut syndrome (LGS) shares many of the features of MAE and is described below. When MAE evolves rapidly with regression of motor and cognitive skills or other movement disorders (specifically ataxia) or both, an underlying neuro-degenerative disease is often suspected. The neuro-degenerative disease most likely to present in this way is late infantile neuronal ceroid lipofuscinosis. Occasionally mitochondrial disorders or other degenerative diseases may also present in this way.

Prolonged absence seizures and non-convulsive status epilepticus lasting hours or days occur relatively commonly in MAE (up to 95% in some series).

The child is usually neurologically normal and has normal neuro-imaging. The EEG demonstrates a normal background with prominent rhythmical theta waves in central regions. There are bursts of generalized spike-wave that may be irregular and may have a frequency of 2–3 cycles/second. During episodes of non-convulsive status epilepticus (NCSE) the spike-wave activity becomes continuous.

The prognosis is variable. Some children will respond to treatment and remain under good control, others will be drug resistant but ultimately the seizures remit, whereas in some the epilepsy remains intractable with severe cognitive and behavioral consequences. In approximately two-thirds of patients, seizures have a self-limiting course.

Lennox–Gastaut syndrome (LGS) is a severe and characteristically refractory epilepsy with multiple seizure types. It shares some features with MAE. Some clinicians do not distinguish between LGS and MAE, and group all severe epilepsies with 'drop attacks,' absences and epileptic encephalopathy together. There are good arguments for keeping them distinct, at least until such time as our understanding of the pathogenesis has advanced and specifically whether genetic markers are identified that may be able to differentiate the two syndromes. There are clearly overlapping features.

The core features of LGS include: multiple seizure types that always include tonic seizures during sleep (and often when awake). Tonic seizures during sleep may be subtle and overlooked. Atypical absences with episodes of non-convulsive status epilepticus are common. Atonic seizures, as manifest by a 'drop attack,' are common and both generalized tonic-clonic and focal seizures may also occur. Myoclonic seizures are not part of the core syndrome but may also occur, either in isolation or before an atonic seizure.

The EEG shows an abnormal background and frequent bursts of slow spike and wave activity at 1–2 cycles/second. The EEG hallmark of tonic seizures is a burst of diffuse rapid spike activity at 10–20Hz. Focal abnormalities may be present.

At least 20% of LGS may evolve from West syndrome. In other situations it is often but not always symptomatic of a severe underlying neurological disorder and neuro-imaging abnormalities are common.

The prognosis of LGS is generally poor. It is one of the most drug resistant epilepsy syndromes and six-month seizure control is rarely achieved and spontaneous remission is very rare ($< 5\%$). All have some degree of learning difficulties and at least 50% show severe cognitive impairment. There is an increased risk of dying prematurely, mainly from any underlying neurological disorder but also in some cases because of sudden unexpected death in epilepsy (SUDEP). For those who survive into adult life, seizure control may improve, but the vast majority cannot live independently.

Symptomatic focal, generalized or neither focal or generalized epilepsies

There are many different neurological disorders (genetic or acquired or both) where epileptic seizures may occur. Some etiologies suggest specific treatments (14) and structural abnormalities may be amenable to surgery.

Magnetic resonance imaging (MRI) is clearly the most useful investigation (15). When seizures are clearly focal, a structural cause should be strongly suspected and actively sought. A structural cause should not be automatically excluded on the basis of a single 'normal' MRI scan.

Issues to consider when imaging is normal in a child with overtly focal seizures
- were the images of adequate quality?
- were the appropriate sequences performed?
- was the imaging reported by a sufficiently expert radiologist?
- was the imaging undertaken at a very young age?
- consider repeating cerebral MRI, particularly if the seizures have definite focal symptomatology, or remain poorly controlled, or both
- consider repeating the MRI scan if the initial scan was undertaken at < 12 months of age; ideally the repeat MRI should be with at least a 1.5 Tesla scanner
- have a very low threshold for referring the child for a specialist pediatric epilepsy opinion

---

Summary

There is a large differential diagnosis for paroxysmal events starting in childhood and misdiagnosis of non-epileptic events as epilepsy, or vice versa, is common. A detailed history from an eye-witness remains the cornerstone of diagnosis. A video recording of the event is often of great additional value. The EEG should not be used as a substitute for an accurate and comprehensive history; it should not be used to 'confirm' or 'exclude' a diagnosis of epilepsy – unless the child has one of their typical clinical events/episodes during the EEG.

Epileptic seizures can present in many different ways and it is important for the clinician to have a working differential diagnosis in mind for each of the major categories of paroxysmal behaviors that occur in this age group.

Investigation is largely directed at determining the etiology of the seizures. The most useful investigation is the MRI scan, which can identify structural abnormalities (genetic or acquired) in an increasing proportion of patients. When the etiology is unclear, and particularly if seizures are poorly controlled, then additional investigations will be necessary. The scope and extent of these investigations will depend on the specific clinical situation. It is particularly important to rule out genetic/metabolic conditions where there might be a specific and non-anticonvulsant treatment.

The concept of the epilepsy syndrome remains useful in clinical practice. A number of syndromes characteristically present in childhood. These include idiopathic syndromes such as childhood absence epilepsy and BECTS, syndromes which are probably idiopathic such as MAE, and syndromes which are more usually symptomatic such as LGS. Many symptomatic epilepsies will present in this age group. However, in many children who have a definite diagnosis of epilepsy, a syndrome diagnosis is not possible and it is important to avoid 'squeezing' such children into a specific syndrome if they do not meet the necessary inclusion criteria.

Management of epilepsy in middle childhood: introduction

This section will focus on the 'middle treatment' of epilepsy in the 2- to 12-year-old range, beginning immediately after the diagnosis, investigation and initiation of antiepileptic medication. Important issues that arise during this time include the most appropriate choice of antiepileptic drug (AED), compliance (concordance) with and monitoring of medication, decisions on appropriate but not excessive restrictions on activity, the recognition and management of co-morbidities including attention and behavior problems, depression and anxiety, cognitive delay, and management issues after failure of initial medication.

Specific antiepileptic drug (AED) treatment will be discussed later in this chapter, and will address the initial, first-line drugs as well as the second-line drugs and most appropriate adjunctive therapy, primarily because there is very limited randomized controlled evidence underpinning the choice of drugs and also because of significant overlap between first- and second-choice drug treatments.

Compliance (concordance) and monitoring of medication

Lack of compliance with medication may result in suboptimal seizure control. In a survey of patients with epilepsy, 71% reported missing occasional doses and almost half reported seizures as a result of missed medication (16).

In order to improve compliance, medication-dosing schedules should be kept as simple as possible. Compliance declines with increasing number of daily doses (16). Ideally, medication should be given no more than twice daily, and scheduled to coincide with regular activities, such as meals, washing/showering in the morning or bedtime. Antiepileptic medication that is ineffective should be withdrawn. While rational polytherapy can be a reasonable therapeutic option, there is rarely any reason to maintain children on more than two (or extremely rarely, three) antiepileptic medications simultaneously on a long-term basis.

The partnership between the doctor and the child (and the family) is integral to maximize compliance, for both attendance in clinic and antiepileptic medication. Children, teenagers and their families should understand what impact further seizures could have, as well as the adverse effects of antiepileptic drugs. Older children or adolescents who have been seizure-free for some time may not fully understand or appreciate the consequences of further seizures and may attempt self-cessation or withdrawal of their medication. Patients will be more likely to take medication as prescribed if they first, believe the treatment is necessary and will help to control seizures, and second, have confidence that they will be monitored closely for side effects. The administration of medication should generally be supervised by an adult through to the early teenage years. Use of a daily or weekly medication (pill or tablet) dispenser may improve compliance with the pills or tablets counted out for each dose ahead of time. This allows care-givers or patients to double-check if the dose has been taken, particularly in busy or chaotic households where more than one person may give the medication, or in situations where the older child is responsible for taking his or her own medication.

Even in the most organized and compliant families, doses will occasionally be missed. In this situation, the missed dose should be given as soon as it is realized. Unless the dose is made up, the blood level may drop and can take five half-lives to recover, leaving the child at increased risk of seizures over this time. Therefore, in most situations, if the missed dose is not recognized until the time of the subsequent dose, the two doses should be taken together; however, this approach is not universal and is not routine practice in the UK. It is never advisable to give a triple dose.

Medication compliance should be addressed at follow-up visits by asking how often doses are missed and the factors leading to the missed doses. Blood levels can theoretically be used to measure compliance, although they are rarely performed specifically for this purpose. Spontaneous variation can be seen with certain medications and levels vary significantly depending on when the blood is taken in relation to the dose of medication. Levels should be measured as trough values. A random blood level undertaken at the time of the clinic consultation may be helpful if it reveals a very low level of or undetectable anticonvulsant; this would suggest either no or very poor compliance with medication. Additional measures of compliance include pill or tablet counts and the use of pill bottles with microprocessors in the caps which record every bottle opening.

In addition to compliance, adverse effects must be enquired about at each visit. Approximately one in eight children who 'fail' their first antiepileptic drug will do so because of adverse effects only (17, 18).

Restrictions

The risk of accidental death in most children with active epilepsy is reassuringly low. In pediatric population-based studies, the accidental death rate in children with epilepsy ranged from 11 to as high as 57 per 100,000 person-years (19) (20). Two other pediatric cohort studies reported a risk of 21 per 100,000 person years (21) and no accidental deaths in 2,360 person-years of follow-up (22).

What appears to be clear is that most deaths in children with epilepsy are the result of their underlying neurological problems, rather than secondary to the seizures themselves (19). However, there are specific safety issues that must be addressed in all children presenting with a first seizure, and reinforced for children with active epilepsy.

Submersion injury

Drowning is a significant risk in all children with active epilepsy, owing to the sudden and unpredictable nature of most seizures. A retrospective, population-based cohort study of all submersion injuries in children and teenagers in a single county in the USA showed a surprisingly high rate in children with epilepsy (23). Those with epilepsy had a relative risk of 13.9 for submersion, and of 13.8 for fatal drowning compared to children without epilepsy, and were more likely to be five years of age or older at time of submersion. The most common sites for submersion were the bath or a swimming pool, with a very high relative risk of 96 for drowning in a bath, and of 23.4 for drowning in a pool. A second survey from the UK found that children with epilepsy were 7.5 times more likely to experience submersion injury or death than those without seizures (24). Nearly all deaths resulted from bathing or swimming unsupervised, although rarely they can occur from a shower when the drain becomes obstructed by the person's body. Consequently, children and teenagers should be supervised at all times when swimming by a responsible adult, who is able to respond immediately at the first sign of a seizure. Simply relying on the on-duty lifeguard is not adequate. Although this may sound excessive and over-restrictive, the supervising adult can usually be unobtrusive. Unless the child is willing to be supervised by an adult while in the bath, showers should be recommended, and the door should be left closed, but unlocked. Hot water temperature should be regulated to minimize the risk of scald injuries.

Other injuries

Burns, fractures, head, dental and soft tissue injuries are only minimally, if at all, increased in most children with epilepsy. However, those with frequent seizures, particularly if seizures result in recurrent falls, are more prone to injury, and require greater supervision. While helmets are frequently prescribed in this population, there is some question as to their efficacy in preventing injuries, and particularly facial injuries (25). Because many of the older antiepileptic drugs (specifically, phenobarbital, phenytoin and sodium valproate) may reduce bone mineral density, it is important to ensure that children treated with these drugs, particularly those with disorders which impair mobilization such as cerebral palsy or degenerative disorders, receive adequate calcium and vitamin D (26).

Children with absence seizures may be at higher risk for bicycle accidents in some (27) but not all studies (28). While most children with epilepsy should be allowed to ride their bicycle provided they wear a helmet, those with frequent absence seizures should probably refrain from this activity until they demonstrate significant seizure control.

Balancing risk of injury and achievement of independence and social growth

Having epilepsy poses inherent challenges to achieving independence and participating fully in social activities, which are obviously important developmental skills in later childhood and adolescence. While some restrictions will be reasonable to protect the child's safety, these may further limit independence, self-empowerment and social development. Parents report disability caused by restrictions in 83% of children with active epilepsy (29). Higher disability was seen in children whose neurologist had recommended at least some restrictions, emphasizing that physicians need to be aware of the impact of their recommendations when they counsel patients. Doctors must also try to ensure that when recommending restrictions, these are, wherever possible, evidence-based and are not simply based on any personal opinion or prejudice.

With rare exceptions, persons with epilepsy should be encouraged to participate in regular physical activity. Contact sports are not precluded, as there is no evidence they induce seizures. Swimming and water sports, harnessed rock climbing, horseback riding and gymnastics are safe with appropriate supervision. However certain sports such as free-climbing, sky diving, hang-gliding and scuba diving could be particularly dangerous if a seizure occurred, and should be avoided in the presence of active, and particularly poorly controlled, epilepsy.

In patients who have had a single seizure, or those weaning antiepileptic medication after achieving seizure freedom, restrictions can be relaxed after 18–24 months, as most seizures would probably have recurred by that time.

Co-morbidities in pediatric epilepsy

Long-term psychosocial outcome is often poor in children with epilepsy, even in those whose seizures eventually spontaneously remit (30–32). The reason for this poor outcome, at least in part, is owing to ongoing co-morbidities. The management of a child with epilepsy goes far beyond the prescription of antiepileptic medication. Children with epilepsy are at high risk for co-morbidities including attention problems, depression, anxiety, poor social skills and sleep disturbances (see Table 3.2). The etiology of these co-morbidities is poorly understood. The

Table 3.2 Types and prevalence of co-morbidities in pediatric epilepsy

Co-morbidity	Approximate prevalence
Cognitive delay	33%
Attention deficit disorder	33%
Behavior problems	29% uncomplicated epilepsy
	58% if associated brain injury
Depression	25%
Anxiety	33%
Psychosis	rare
Sleep disturbance	Approximately 33–50%

observation that many of these co-morbidities pre-date the onset of seizures would suggest that they cannot be fully explained by either the neurological or psychological consequence and impact of frequent seizures. This might suggest that they are, in part, a result of altered neurotransmitters or the cerebral substrate which also predispose to epilepsy, rather than just simply the result of the seizures themselves.

The under-recognition of co-morbidities remains a significant problem in children with epilepsy. The use of screening instruments would be ideal to identify any associated difficulties (as in concentration, memory or processing impairments) but, at a minimum, physicians should ask families about any concerns in these areas as part of the child's routine care. There is often hesitation to introduce additional and different medications (such as stimulants or anti-depressants) in children with epilepsy. However, the under-treatment of these conditions may potentially worsen the child's quality of life, may impair achievement of academic goals (and educational and employment potential) and can result in a less favorable long-term psychosocial outcome. Furthermore, failure to address these co-morbidities often results in multiple changes in antiepileptic medication or doses, or both, because these drugs are often blamed for behavior problems.

Cognitive delay

Intellectual disability affects nearly one-third of children with epilepsy (33). In a cohort of children with established epilepsy caused by a range of epilepsy syndromes, including idiopathic generalized epilepsy, Nolan *et al.* found that intellectual ability generally fell below the normal range; clearly, this is difficult to interpret and equally difficult to generalize for all children with epilepsy, given the heterogeneity of the different syndromes reported in this study, but the findings cannot be ignored (34). Cognitive disability is not only a concern for children with underlying structural brain lesions or chronic, intractable seizures, but may be present early in the course of epilepsy. Significantly poorer performance in intelligence, language, executive function and psychomotor speed was found in children with newly diagnosed epilepsy who were otherwise neurologically and developmentally normal and who had normal brain magnetic resonance imaging (35). While a number of studies have addressed whether cognitive function deteriorates over time and have shown a range of results, there is some evidence that cognitive decline is progressive, especially in those with more severe epilepsy (36). In addition, a recent prospective study suggests that the presence of neuro-behavioral co-morbidities (cognitive problems or attention deficit) at onset of epilepsy is predictive of abnormal, longer-term cognitive impairments (37).

Attention deficit disorder and behavior problems

Epidemiologic studies using standardized scales have demonstrated between a two- and almost six-fold increased incidence of attention deficit hyperactivity disorder (ADHD) in children with epilepsy (38, 39). Whereas most children without epilepsy have the combined subtype of ADHD, two studies have found a high prevalence of the inattentive subtype in children with epilepsy (38, 39). Attention and behavior problems have been found to be present even prior to the first seizure (40) and may be progressive (41).

Only a few studies have evaluated whether specific epilepsy variables predispose to a higher likelihood of ADHD. Dunn *et al.* found no significant factors from the type or severity of epilepsy that were able to predict the risk of ADHD; however, there was a trend for the inattentive subtype to occur more frequently in children with absence and partial complex seizures and the combined subtype to occur more often in those with generalized convulsive seizures (38). A recent study found that lower IQ scores correlated with higher prevalence of ADHD in children with a new or a recent onset of idiopathic epilepsy; however, the epilepsy type, number of AEDs, duration of epilepsy or age at seizure onset did not (39). Epilepsy severity may be a specific risk factor. Another study observed that over 60% of children with severe epilepsy met screening criteria for ADHD (42). In this population, the combined subtype was more prevalent in children with earlier onset of epilepsy, generalized epilepsy and lower adaptive level, while the inattentive subtype occurred more often in those with focal (partial) epilepsy.

Stimulant medications are the primary therapeutic agent for treatment of ADHD, but under-treatment of these symptoms in children with co-morbid ADHD and epilepsy remains a significant problem (39). A recent 'expert opinion' on the use of methylphenidate in children with epilepsy documents significant improvement in ADHD symptoms without exacerbation of seizures or an adverse effect on serum antiepileptic drug levels (43).

Behavior problems are also more prevalent in children with epilepsy. In a seminal and large prevalence study, mental health problems were demonstrated in 29% of children with uncomplicated seizures, and in 58% of children with both seizures and brain damage, compared to only 7% of the general population (44). Again, behavior problems seem to develop early in the course of epilepsy, and are likely pre-date seizure onset. Predictably, poor seizure control and underlying neurological dysfunction seem to correlate with higher rates of behavior problems (44).

Depression and anxiety

Depression and anxiety have also been found to have a higher prevalence in children with epilepsy and often become manifest early in the course, even pre-dating seizure onset. In a study of children and teenagers with new-onset, idiopathic epilepsy, almost one quarter were found to have a depressive disorder and over one-third had an anxiety disorder, based on a structured psychiatric diagnostic interview (45). In children and teenagers with established epilepsy who had significantly elevated scores on depression or anxiety scales, none was noted to have been diagnosed previously with a mood disorder, suggesting that these disorders in children with epilepsy are poorly recognized and consequently are likely to go untreated (46).

Psychosis

Psychosis is, fortunately, rare in pediatric epilepsy (47). Rarely, a post-ictal psychosis may be seen but usually resolves spontaneously after a few days. Many antiepileptic drugs have been reported to induce psychotic reactions on rare occasions, particularly gabapentin, topiramate and vigabatrin and less commonly, levetiracetam.

Sleep

In children with epilepsy, sleep may be disrupted as a result of the underlying brain abnormality, nocturnal seizures, paroxysmal EEG abnormalities, side effects of antiepileptic medication, impaired release of melatonin and parent or child anxiety, or a combination of a number of these factors. Sleep disorders appear to be more prevalent in children with epilepsy than healthy controls (48, 49). Refractory epilepsy, higher seizure-frequency, remote symptomatic etiology and associated developmental delay all correlate with impaired sleep. In addition, obstructive sleep apnea may be more common in those with epilepsy and its treatment may correlate with significant improvement in seizure control (50). Predictably, children with more pronounced sleep disruption appear to be at greater risk of developing behavior problems.

Autism

Approximately 30% of children with 'typical' (primary) autism will ultimately develop epilepsy (51). This shows a bimodal age distribution, with a peak age of seizure onset in the preschool years or around puberty. Children with greater severity of learning difficulties (mental handicap) or autism, those with overt motor deficits and those with regression developing after three years of age are at higher risk of seizures. Genetic disorders, including ring chromosome 20, Down's, Angelman, Rett or Smith–Magenis syndrome, tuberous sclerosis and neurofibromatosis type I are also associated with a greater risk of epilepsy.

There is also a greater risk of certain populations of children with early-onset epilepsy developing autistic spectrum disorders (ASD). Infants with West syndrome, particularly those with tuberous sclerosis and a temporal lobe tuber, or those in whom the diagnosis (or effective therapy) has been delayed are at particular risk of developing ASD.

The possibility of continuous spike-wave in slow-sleep (CSWSS) with the clinical correlate being electrical status epilepticus during slow-wave sleep (ESESS), must be considered in those children with epilepsy who appear to regress, and particularly in receptive and expressive language and social skills. These children should undergo an overnight EEG recording; an outpatient sleeping EEG may not allow the child to enter the deeper stages of sleep to confirm (or refute) CSWSS.

Antiepileptic medication; what to do if the first antiepileptic drug fails?

Ensure compliance and re-evaluate the diagnosis and epilepsy syndrome

Failure of the first antiepileptic drug for lack of efficacy occurs in approximately one quarter of children (52, 53). If a first drug fails for lack of efficacy, the clinician should review if the child's medication is being taken in the prescribed dose and that compliance (concordance) is consistent and good. Next, the diagnosis of epilepsy, the seizure type and epilepsy syndrome should be reviewed to ensure their accuracy. Misdiagnosis of epilepsy is common, being reported in 23% in a population-based study and in 30% of a cohort of children referred to a tertiary epilepsy centre (54). Inaccurate diagnosis may result in medical harm (if a diagnosis such as hypoglycemia or a cardiac arrhythmia is missed or if the child develops an adverse effect to an antiepileptic drug), or psychosocial harm (if the child is subjected to restricted sports or social activities owing to concerns about seizures, or if a child's psychogenic non-epileptic seizures caused by physical or sexual abuse is not recognized).

The epilepsy syndrome should also be defined wherever possible to ensure medication choices are appropriate and will not exacerbate seizures. Carbamazepine has been the most implicated antiepileptic drug in seizure exacerbation and is contraindicated in the presence of generalized spike and wave activity, as it may aggravate both typical and atypical absence, myoclonic and atonic seizures and may provoke non-convulsive status epilepticus (55, 56). It may also worsen myoclonus in the progressive myoclonic epilepsies and Angelman syndrome. Aggravation of benign epilepsy of childhood with centro-temporal spikes leading to either CSWSS (or ESESS) or epileptic negative myoclonus has been reported (57, 58), and the drug is contraindicated in Landau–Kleffner syndrome. Studies have also documented worsening of other partial seizures (55). Exacerbation of epileptic discharges (specifically spike and wave activity) in the EEG following the introduction of carbamazepine predicts increased risk of seizure exacerbation (55, 56).

Table 3.3 Expert opinion regarding first-line medication for pediatric epilepsy

Epilepsy syndrome	US expert opinion	European expert opinion
Idiopathic partial	Oxcarbazepine, carbamazepine, gabapentin, lamotrigine, levetiracetam	Valproic acid (sodium valproate)*
Cryptogenic or symptomatic partial	Oxcarbazepine, carbamazepine, levetiracetam, lamotrigine	Carbamazepine, oxcarbazepine, valproic acid
Idiopathic generalized	Ethosuximide (only for childhood absence epilepsy), valproic acid, lamotrigine	Ethosuximide (only for childhood absence epilepsy), valproic acid, lamotrigine
Symptomatic generalized	Valproic acid, lamotrigine, topiramate	Valproic acid, lamotrigine, topiramate

* Some European experts would recommend carbamazepine or lamotrigine.

Vigabatrin is contraindicated in absence epilepsy and may induce non-convulsive status epilepticus and may also exacerbate myoclonic seizures (59); this emphasizes the importance of the correct differentiation of myoclonic seizures from infantile spasms, both of which are common seizure types in infancy. Tiagabine is also known to worsen absence epilepsy and may induce absence status and is now rarely prescribed for most of the pediatric epilepsies. In Lennox–Gastaut syndrome, gabapentin has been shown to aggravate atypical absences and myoclonic seizures. Intravenous benzodiazepines given to treat absence status may also rarely precipitate tonic status epilepticus in Lennox–Gastaut syndrome (60).

How to choose the next most appropriate antiepileptic drug

In theory, it may be reasonable to consider the mechanism of action, as it makes little sense to prescribe (and there is little evidence to support this) a second drug with a very similar mechanism of action as the first drug, if the first failed because of lack of efficacy. The choice of which treatment to use is dependent on clinical judgment, and 'expert opinions' have been published from both the US and Europe (61, 62). (See Table 3.3.)

a. Idiopathic generalized epilepsy

First-line antiepileptic drugs for treatment of idiopathic generalized epilepsy include valproic acid (sodium valproate), lamotrigine and ethosuximide (although the latter is only of use in childhood absence epilepsy or occasionally in absences with myoclonus). A recent study compared these three drugs in the treatment of children with newly diagnosed childhood-onset absence epilepsy and found a higher response rate with either ethosuximide or valproic acid (sodium valproate) compared to lamotrigine (63).

If one of these agents fails to control seizures, or leads to unacceptable adverse effects, or both, it should be replaced by another of these first-choice drugs. Although ethosuximide is efficacious for absence seizures it has no effect on generalized tonic-clonic seizures; it is therefore not an appropriate drug for juvenile absence or juvenile myoclonic epilepsy, given the much higher incidence of tonic-clonic seizures in these syndromes. While valproic acid is very effective for suppressing many generalized seizures, it may be associated with weight gain, menstrual irregularities and polycystic ovary syndrome in adolescent women and if taken early in pregnancy, may result in neural tube and other congenital abnormalities in the fetus, or developmental (and specifically communication) problems in the schoolchild exposed to sodium valproate in utero. In view of these potential concerns, many, but not all, clinicians will try other medications prior to using it in teenagers and women of childbearing age or potential. It is important to give the parents and teenager the facts and correct information about the different antiepileptic drug options so that they are able to make an informed decision in their management. If valproic acid is used in this population, folic acid should also be prescribed, in a recommended dose of 5 mg per day. Other antiepileptic drugs which may be effective in idiopathic generalized epilepsy include levetiracetam, topiramate, zonisamide and clobazam and, to a far lesser extent, felbamate and acetazolamide.

b. Symptomatic generalized epilepsy

These epilepsy syndromes are, as a rule, more refractory to treatment. Lamotrigine, topiramate, felbamate and most recently rufinamide (64) have been shown to be more effective than placebo in controlled trials in children with Lennox–Gastaut syndrome (65). The role of rufinamide may be limited to its efficacy in treating 'drop' seizures, an umbrella term for different seizure types, including myoclonic, tonic and atonic. Felbamate may be helpful, but is prescribed infrequently, particularly in the UK. Given the potential for aplastic anemia and liver failure, felbamate should be reserved for genuinely severe and refractory cases. Valproic acid is also felt to be effective, although it has never been studied in a randomized, placebo-controlled trial. While lamotrigine can be effective, its slow titration limits its use in children experiencing very frequent seizures. In addition, high doses (>10 mg/kg/day) may occasionally result in a paradoxical deterioration in seizure control. In addition, lamotrigine may also result in a marked exacerbation of both convulsive and myoclonic aseizures in SMEI (Dravet syndrome). First-line drugs are generally considered to be valproic acid, lamotrigine or topiramate. If one drug fails, another in this group, or clobazam, could be prescribed. Clobazam and topiramate demonstrate a relatively broad spectrum of action, and may therefore be useful in a number of epilepsy syndromes and epilepsies, including the Lennox–Gastaut syndrome and severe myoclonic epilepsy of infancy (SMEI, Dravet syndrome) and genetic syndromes such as Angelman and Rett syndromes. Rufinamide, in combination with sodium valproate, may be particularly useful in Lennox–Gastaut syndrome. Zonisamide and levetiracetam may also be useful alternatives. The potential danger in these groups of children is excessive polypharmacy – simply adding one or more drugs without withdrawing another antiepileptic drug; one must never lose sight of the overall functioning of the child in attempting to control their seizures.

The ketogenic diet can be very effective in many cases. Different variants of the diet are available – 'classical,' 'medium chain triglyceride (MCT)' or the modified Atkins diet – but all demand relatively strict adherence and may be poorly tolerated by the children and may cause significant gastrointestinal side effects (constipation or diarrhea) (66, 67). Both the child and the family need to be well motivated and need to be supported by an adequately trained and resourced team. Discontinuation of the ketogenic diet because of gastrointestinal side effects or poor compliance is almost as common as stopping because of lack of efficacy; in addition, an initial good response to the diet may be lost after a number of months, even years, for no obvious reason.

Idiopathic partial epilepsy

The seizures in both early-onset benign occipital epilepsy and benign epilepsy of childhood with centro-temporal (rolandic) spikes are usually infrequent and if treatment is needed, generally respond well to medication. The antiepileptic drugs used in partial epilepsy are quite effective with 50% to 65% of patients having no further seizures once medication is started. Carbamazepine (or oxcarbazepine), lamotrigine, levetiracetam and gabapentin are frequently used in idiopathic partial epilepsy, given their low potential for adverse effects, although gabapentin may be associated with behavioral side effects, thereby limiting its use. However, only sulthiame has been shown to be more efficacious than placebo in the treatment of benign epilepsy with centro-temporal spikes (68). Sulthiame is rarely used in the UK, in contrast to some European countries and, to a lesser extent, the US and Canada. A similar study (published in abstract form only) using gabapentin in the same epilepsy syndrome failed to show statistically significant benefit, although a trend for improvement was seen. While carbamazepine or oxcarbazepine are usually associated with seizure control, these drugs can rarely exacerbate epileptic discharges resulting in electrical status epilepticus of slow-wave sleep (ESESS), with regression in language, cognitive skills and/or executive functioning.

Symptomatic partial epilepsy

Numerous antiepileptic drugs may be effective in these epilepsies. The choice of first-line therapy is usually dictated by its side effect profile with the most common choices being carbamazepine, oxcarbazepine, levetiracetam, clobazam or valproate. If adult experience is confirmed in children, lacosamide may also prove to be a useful drug, given its ease of use, very few side effects, although dizziness may be a significant problem particularly in higher doses; it also appears to have little or even no recognized drug interactions. There is little evidence that one particular agent is more efficacious than another. A second antiepileptic medication with low potential for toxicity should be tried if the first fails, prior to considering surgical therapy, unless the child has a clear, potentially progressive, structural lesion in which case surgery should be considered much earlier. Once again, polypharmacy becomes a real temptation in this group of patients, given the long list of antiepileptic drugs that could be prescribed; therefore the clinician's mantra should be, 'If I add, I must take away!'

Later management of epilepsy in middle childhood: introduction

This section focuses on the 'later treatment' of epilepsy in the 2- to 12-year old range. In many children, seizure freedom is achieved and the issues of duration of treatment, when and how to withdraw antiepileptic medication and risk of recurrence will be reviewed. However, some children will demonstrate a much more difficult course and will respond incompletely or poorly to medication. Treatment options for this group, include further antiepileptic drugs, dietary and other therapies, and surgery, either resective or palliative. Finally, the long-term medical, cognitive and social prognosis of children with epilepsy will be reviewed, with specific emphasis on epilepsy syndromes.

What is the duration of treatment with an antiepileptic drug?

Most children who achieve one- or two-year seizure freedom on antiepileptic therapy will remain seizure-free after it has been discontinued. Consequently, the continued use of antiepileptic drugs in children who have been seizure-free for five or more years is probably unnecessary. The decision as to when to attempt withdrawal of medication must be made together with the child and family, taking into account the likely risk of recurrence, but also the impact of further seizures on education, social (leisure activities), emotional and personal well-being. However, in seizure-free children, it is generally easier to wean medication prior to adolescence, when issues such as driving and career choices make this decision more complex.

The duration of seizure freedom prior to withdrawal of medication has been assessed in a few studies. A review of this topic found evidence to support a seizure-free period of at least two years in children with an abnormal EEG and partial seizures; however, there was insufficient evidence to guide duration of therapy in children with generalized seizures and normal EEGs (69). Those with easily controlled seizures may also not require two years of therapy. In one study of children who became seizure-free within two months of starting antiepileptic medication, and who remained seizure-free, there was no difference in relapse rate when withdrawal of medication occurred after six months compared to after 12 months (70).

The optimal duration of therapy in benign childhood epilepsy with centrotemporal spikes has not been resolved. Many children continue to show epileptic discharges despite having no further seizures. The decision to withdraw medication should not be based on the absence of EEG discharges but on the natural history of this syndrome. A relatively old study showed that approximately half of children remit by age six years, and approximately 90% remit by age twelve years (71). As such, one to two years of treatment seems reasonable for younger children. Most children over the age of eight years will not relapse even when medications are withdrawn after only one year of seizure freedom.

The decision to wean medication in patients who have achieved seizure freedom following epilepsy surgery remains controversial. There are no clear data indicating when an antiepileptic drug can be withdrawn, although most clinicians would attempt this in children who have been seizure-free for between six and 12 months following resective surgery.

In non-surgical cases, most clinicians will usually continue medication for a minimum of two years of seizure freedom before considering drug withdrawal. Seizures will recur in up to one-third of patients, although the precise rate of recurrence will depend on the epilepsy syndrome and cause of the epilepsy.

What is the risk of relapse?

This important topic is addressed in detail in Chapter 5. Approximately 60–70% of children whose seizures are controlled for one to three years will remain seizure-free when medication is withdrawn. Most patients who relapse do so either during the withdrawal (weaning) period or within the first year after medication has been discontinued. Reassuringly, the vast majority of children who relapse after discontinuation of antiepileptic drugs regain seizure control when medication is reinstituted, and only 1–5% subsequently develop intractable epilepsy (72).

How should medication be withdrawn?

In seizure-free patients receiving more than one antiepileptic drug, medications should be weaned one at a time. The first drug to be stopped is generally the one considered least efficacious or the most associated with side effects. There is little evidence to guide the rapidity of medication taper (73), but most clinicians taper over a minimum of one month and a maximum of three months. The recurrence of seizures during the withdrawal period should prompt re-initiation of medication. Withdrawal is often, and entirely arbitrarily, undertaken more gradually if a child has been receiving phenobarbital or a benzodiazepine for a number of years.

What should be done if seizures persist?

Approximately 25–30% of children with epilepsy are medically intractable. There is no universal definition of 'intractable,' but pragmatically this usually implies that the child continues to experience ongoing seizures despite having received at least two appropriate antiepileptic drugs. Intractable epilepsy places the child at risk of physical injury, learning and cognitive disability, social embarrassment, inability to achieve independence, unemployment, inability to drive, the effects of polypharmacy, and it may have a major detrimental impact on family life and the development of personal relationships. Early, accurate identification of intractability is important to allow evaluation for possible epilepsy surgery or other

Table 3.4 Epilepsies or epilepsy syndromes with apparent unique response to specific antiepileptic drugs

Syndrome	Medication
West syndrome caused by tuberous sclerosis	Vigabatrin
Severe myoclonic epilepsy of infancy (Dravet syndrome)	Stiripentol used in combination with valproate and/or clobazam
Atypical benign partial epilepsy of childhood and some cases of idiopathic Landau–Kleffner syndrome	Sulthiame
Progressive myoclonic epilepsies	Piracetam
Continuous spike-wave of slow-wave sleep (CSWSS)	Prednisolone; high-dose clobazam

alternative treatments, to avoid the adverse effects of ineffective medications and to improve long-term quality of life. However, there are risks from surgery and the diagnosis of medical intractability must be accurate. One of the most robust predictors of medical intractability in children is the specific epilepsy syndrome. After two years of follow-up, medical intractability was present in 56% with symptomatic generalized epilepsy, 13% with symptomatic localization-related epilepsy, but only 2–3% with idiopathic generalized or partial epilepsy (74). Therapeutic options in these patients include further trials of antiepileptic drugs or other medical therapies (corticosteroids and, rarely, intravenous immuno-globulins), the ketogenic diet, resective epilepsy surgery or palliative surgical procedures (vagal nerve stimulation or corpus callosotomy).

Further trials of antiepileptic medication

The chance of successful seizure control diminishes with increasing numbers of antiepileptic medications. In a prospective survey of all children with epilepsy, after failing three antiepileptic drugs for lack of efficacy, only 10% responded favorably to another medication (75). The prognosis for children with focal (partial) epilepsy is of more concern. In one study, only 29% who did not respond to their first antiepileptic drug became seizure-free on a different monotherapy (76), and in another study, seizure control was achieved in only 11% after failing two drugs (77). While there are certain epilepsy syndromes which may show unique efficacy to specific medications (Table 3.4), these syndromes constitute only a very small portion of children with intractable epilepsy. In general, children who fail to respond to two appropriate antiepileptic medications at therapeutic doses should be considered for a surgical or dietary therapy.

Resective surgery

This topic is also addressed in detail in Chapter 4. Children with non-idiopathic, focal (partial or localization-related) epilepsy who have a probable single seizure focus based on seizure semiology (detailed description of the seizure) or prior EEG data, and who have failed two (or at most three) appropriate antiepileptic medications at therapeutic doses for lack of efficacy should be considered for a surgical evaluation. This is because it is unlikely that additional antiepileptic drug therapy will control seizures. Cortical dysplasia and perinatal brain injuries are probably the most common pathologies identified in children undergoing surgery for intractable epilepsy; however, other potentially resectable lesions include mesial temporal sclerosis, tumors, neuro-cutaneous disorders, postnatally acquired lesions, vascular malformations, hemimegalencephaly or Rasmussen's syndrome. Dual pathology is more common in children and refers to the co-existence of mesial temporal sclerosis with an additional lesion including cortical dysplasia, a neuro-cutaneous syndrome or a tumor. Extra-temporal (typically frontal) and neocortical temporal resections predominate, in contrast to adults where mesial temporal resection is most common. The primary aims of surgical evaluation are to determine first, the definitive epileptogenic zone and second, if this zone contains 'eloquent' cortex, which would result in a post-operative motor or language deficit following resection of this area. The initial pre-surgical evaluation or workup includes recording of several of the child's stereotypic seizures by scalp video–EEG, careful review of cerebral MRI done using specific seizure protocol sequences, consideration of functional brain imaging (functional MRI, single photon emission computed tomography [SPECT] or positron emission tomography [PET]) or magnetoencephalography (MEG), particularly in MRI-negative cases. Ideally MRI should be undertaken using a 3.0 Tesla scanner. Many, if not most children should also undergo neuro-psychological evaluation and, in specific situations, a psychiatric assessment. This initial evaluation will exclude patients with a multifocal onset to their seizures and helps localize the focus in those with a single seizure onset. If the focus can be clearly identified and does not involve eloquent cortex, the child may be able to progress to resection. However, invasive EEG monitoring is often performed in children in the following situations:

- in MRI-negative (non-lesional) cases where the scalp EEG recording can identify the region, but not the precise site of seizure onset
- if the epileptogenic zone appears more widespread than the structural lesion
- when there is non- or dis-concordance of seizure semiology, ictal EEG, functional or structural imaging data
- in selected cases, where there are multiple lesions (as in tuberous sclerosis or where there is obvious dual pathology)
- if the epileptogenic zone is close to eloquent cortex then stimulation-mapping will be needed to identify what motor or language (or both) function may be lost if the lesion is removed (resected).

Outcomes are generally favorable (Table 3.5) (78) but depend on the type and location of surgery, whether a lesion is clearly identifiable on the MRI and completeness of resection. Children with cortical dysplasia often do less well because these lesions may be more extensive than can be seen on MRI, even with higher-resolution scans (3.0 Tesla or even 5.0 Tesla scans) and are more likely to involve eloquent cortex, thereby limiting the margins of the resection.

Table 3.5 Outcome after resective surgery for epilepsy in children

Type of Surgery	Seizure Freedom
Temporal lobectomy	58–78%
Neocortical resection	
-temporal	60–91%
-extratemporal (most commonly, frontal)	54–66%
Hemispherectomy	43–79% (possibly higher in Rasmussen's syndrome)

Palliative surgical procedures

a. Vagal nerve stimulation

Vagal nerve stimulation (VNS) could be considered in patients with intractable epilepsy who are either not suitable surgical candidates or who would have either a low chance of benefit or a high chance of an irreversible deficit from a cortical resection. Although VNS is widely undertaken in children, the data for its efficacy are based predominantly on retrospective case series. There are as yet no randomized controlled trials that have evaluated VNS versus antiepileptic drugs (or other therapies) in children.

Multiple case series have suggested that up to half of children experience a greater than 50% reduction in seizures and up to one-third may experience a greater than 90% reduction (79–81). However, seizure freedom is very rare. In addition, the use of the magnet (to 'swipe' over the stimulator) may reduce seizure duration or intensity, or even abort the seizure in nearly half of cases. Vagal nerve stimulation has been used mostly in symptomatic partial epilepsy, but may also be beneficial in symptomatic generalized epilepsy (82). While a retrospective study reported improvements both in seizure control and in quality of life in children with autism, this has been disputed in a more recent and small prospective study.

b. Corpus callosotomy

Corpus callosotomy is usually considered in cases of symptomatic generalized epilepsy with intractable tonic or atonic seizures resulting in 'drop attacks' or sudden falls, and where neither focal resection nor VNS are considered appropriate. The theory is that dividing this structure will prevent bilateral synchrony of the presumed focal epileptic discharge and thus lessen either the frequency or severity of the seizures. Most surgical centers opt for section of the anterior two-thirds of the corpus callosum, followed by section of the posterior third if seizure control remains poor. However, in children with very poor neurological function, it may be reasonable to perform a complete corpus callosotomy as the initial procedure. Acute disconnection syndrome is a common but often transient complication and includes decreased speech output, apraxia, inattention and incontinence. In the vast majority of patients, these symptoms improve markedly over days to weeks. Long-term complications include sensory dissociation, language dysfunction, hemispheric competition and disorders of attention–memory sequencing. Predictably, these symptoms are more pronounced after complete versus anterior two-thirds callosotomy. It is worth emphasizing that these symptoms may be barely recognizable in the population in whom corpus callosotomy is undertaken because most will have moderate, severe or even profound learning difficulties.

Outcome is highly dependent on seizure type; however between 60 and 83% of children experience a significant reduction in the seizures which cause the child to 'drop' or fall. The reduction in falls may have a marked benefit on quality of life for these patients and their families and may easily outweigh the potential complications including the neuro-psychological effects outlined previously. Partial seizures are not generally improved, and may worsen.

c. Multiple subpial transection

Multiple subpial transection (MST) has been considered where the epileptogenic zone involves eloquent cortex and resection is not possible. Parallel slices are made in the cortex which disrupt horizontal cortical synchronizing networks (and therefore disrupt or prevent seizure propagation), but do not affect subcortical–cortical input. MST probably has only a very limited role, and specifically in treating some children with the Landau–Kleffner syndrome or around the margins of a focal resection, to try and preserve cortical function.

Ketogenic diet

The basis and role of the ketogenic diet has been outlined in detail in Chapter 2 (83).

A recent, randomized controlled trial proved the efficacy of the diet but did not find a significant difference in efficacy between symptomatic generalized and symptomatic focal epilepsy (84). While the diet is most frequently used in young children, patients from infancy to adulthood have sustained benefit. The ketogenic diet is considered the therapy of choice in children with glucose transporter (GLUT-1) deficiency and pyruvate dehydrogenase deficiency, and may also be effective in some forms of mitochondrial disease. It is also an effective treatment option for Lennox–Gastaut syndrome, myoclonic–astatic epilepsy (Doose syndrome), severe myoclonic epilepsy of infancy (Dravet syndrome) and tuberous sclerosis, and should be considered early in the course of these disorders and probably after two antiepileptic drugs have failed to produce any significant or sustained seizure control.

Protocols for initiation of the ketogenic diet vary among centers. Many initiate the diet on an inpatient basis, particularly in children under three years of age. Most centers no longer require an initial fast. Prior to commencing the diet, disorders of fatty acid transport and oxidation, and pyruvate carboxylase deficiency must be ruled out by measurement of carnitine, acylcarnitine, urine organic acids and lactate. The diet should be started in a centre with both a dietician and a physician who are experienced in its use. Patients require supplementation with multivitamins and minerals, and calcium with vitamin D. Children on the diet need to avoid medications and creams or other products with more than minimal amounts of carbohydrate. Lower carbohydrate preparations of medication should be used, which generally will exclude suspensions or chew-tablets. Both the Charlie Foundation in the US (www.charliefoundation.org) and Matthews Friends in the UK (www.matthewsfriends.org) websites are easily accessible by parents and provide valuable information on the diet, including carbohydrate content of various over-the-counter products and a wide range of recipes. If tolerated, a trial of the diet should be given for a minimum of two months. Urinary ketones, and occasionally blood-ketone monitoring will be required by the family. While some achieve good seizure control with only modest levels of ketosis, many children appear to require ketones in the high range.

Regular follow-up is required to monitor efficacy and adverse effects, which include vomiting, constipation, diarrhea, abdominal pain, hyperlipidemia, hyperuricemia, hypocalcemia, acidosis, renal calculi (particularly if the child is also receiving topiramate or zonisamide), cardiomyopathy and poor growth. If the diet is effective, many patients are able to reduce the numbers of antiepileptic drugs; however, most children will still need to remain on one antiepileptic drug, as well as the diet.

Approximately half of children experience a 50% or greater reduction and 20–30% have a greater than 90% reduction in seizures on the diet. In responders, weaning of the diet is often considered after two years by gradual reduction of the ketogenic ratio and return to a normal diet over two to three months.

Other medical options

a. Corticosteroids (85, 86)

In epilepsy during the childhood years (and obviously excluding West syndrome), steroids are most often considered in two clinical situations:
1. electrical status epilepticus of slow-wave sleep (ESESS)
2. an epileptic encephalopathy with a rapidly deteriorating course.

No randomized studies have been undertaken in ESESS to inform clinicians on the dose or duration of therapy; however, many recommend high doses of steroids for fairly prolonged periods. Steroids have been shown to be effective and subsequent work has shown that prednisone (2–5 mg/kg/day), methylprednisolone (20 mg/kg/day for three days) and ACTH or tetracosactide (80 IU/day with a three-month taper) are effective in improving both the EEG abnormality and neuro-psychological function (87). It has been suggested that the earlier steroids are started, the shorter the duration required and the better the outcome. Tapering of steroid may be associated with relapse of ESESS and neuro-psychological deterioration, necessitating longer treatment duration in many children.

Several reports have also noted benefit with steroid therapy in children with symptomatic generalized epilepsy (85, 86). Steroids may be beneficial in cases where the child is clearly deteriorating despite trials of conventional antiepileptic drugs, or is in non-convulsive status epilepticus. No studies have determined which seizure types are more likely to respond and the data cannot provide clear recommendations regarding which type of steroid should be used, in what dose and for how long. The disadvantage of ACTH (tetracosactide) is that it has to be given by intramuscular injection, which is painful and may be associated with local complications. While response rates are favorable, most patients relapse within months or even after steroids are withdrawn. High-dose corticosteroid therapy has also been used in Rasmussen's syndrome. Although seizure frequency may be reduced in the short term, this therapy does not provide long-term stability (88). Clearly, corticosteroids must be used with caution, particularly if used for longer than six weeks, because of the risk of immunosuppression, hypertension and glucose intolerance.

b. Intravenous immunoglobulin (IVIG)

One very small case series has documented that IVIG may be beneficial in Landau–Kleffner syndrome. Two of five newly diagnosed children given IVIG (2 g/kg/day for 4 days) showed resolution of severe language and EEG abnormalities (89).

While case series of children with Lennox–Gastaut syndrome treated with IVIG report that 50–87% have significant improvement, a small add-on, placebo-controlled, single-blind, crossover study was less optimistic (90). In this study, 10 children with Lennox–Gastaut syndrome received either placebo or IVIG (two doses of 400 mg/kg given two weeks apart). The wash-out period was 4 weeks and the total observation time was only 14 weeks. Only two of the ten (20%) showed an immediate reduction in seizure activity and improvement in their EEG, while the remaining eight showed no change.

Although there is a suggestion that IVIG may have a role in the management of both ESESS and symptomatic generalized epilepsy, no recommendations can be made because of very limited data, short follow-up periods, different dose regimens and, in most studies, lack of placebo controls and blinding. Finally, IVIG is in short supply globally, is expensive and carries a small risk of infection from blood-derived products. It is possible, though perhaps unrealistic to expect, that further double-blind, placebo-controlled studies may help to inform clinicians on the role, doses and duration of IVIG therapy.

Finally, IVIG has also been used in Rasmussen's syndrome and may be associated with a transient halt in progression of the neurological deterioration; this may provide useful, but temporary, seizure control prior to hemispherectomy, which is the treatment of choice for children with this progressive disorder.

Prognosis

Medical

A number of factors help to predict the medical outcome of epilepsy in childhood (Table 3.6). One of the strongest predictors is the epilepsy syndrome. Children

Table 3.6 Summary of predictors of intractability

Consistently reported in studies	Inconsistently reported in studies
Seizure frequency or type	**History**
• High initial seizure frequency	• History of febrile seizures (complex > simple)
• Partial seizures; multiple seizure types; atonic or tonic seizures	• History of status epilepticus
• Neonatal or seizures occurring <12 months of age	**Investigations**
• Age of onset >12 years	• Epileptic discharges on EEG
Epilepsy syndrome	• Focal slowing on EEG
• Symptomatic generalized epilepsy	
• Catastrophic epilepsies (some authors use the term 'epileptic encephalopathies')	
Etiology	
• Non-idiopathic	
Physical examination	
• Developmental delay (usually moderate or severe)	
• Neurological deficit	
Investigations	
• MRI showing hippocampal atrophy or hippocampal sclerosis	
• MRI showing cortical dysplasia	
Response to treatment	
• Failure to respond within first year	
• Failure to respond to first antiepileptic drug	

with early-onset benign occipital epilepsy or benign childhood epilepsy with centro-temporal spikes nearly always achieve remission and can ultimately discontinue antiepileptic medication. In those with cryptogenic or symptomatic partial epilepsy, long-term outcome is more difficult to predict with accuracy (91, 92).

Factors which have been reported to correlate with a higher risk of intractability include:

• a history of neonatal seizures
• high initial seizure frequency
• multiple seizure types
• abnormal neurological findings
• developmental delay
• remote symptomatic etiology
• abnormal neuro-imaging with cortical dysplasia or mesial temporal sclerosis
• failure to respond to the first antiepileptic drug.

Approximately two-thirds of children with childhood absence epilepsy (CAE) will enter long-term remission of epilepsy and be able to discontinue antiepileptic drugs (93). However, nearly half of those who fail to remit will ultimately evolve into juvenile myoclonic epilepsy. Juvenile absence epilepsy is less well studied but spontaneous remission is less likely than in CAE and antiepileptic therapy is needed long term to maintain seizure freedom; a significant number of these individuals will subsequently develop tonic-clonic seizures by the late teenage years or early adult life.

Only one population-based study has addressed seizure outcome in symptomatic generalized epilepsy (94). After 18–26 years of follow-up, terminal remission was seen in none of the children with Lennox–Gastaut syndrome, in 56% of those with myoclonic–astatic epilepsy and in 31% of undefined symptomatic generalized epilepsy.

Cognitive

Long-term cognitive outcome is dependent on both cognitive functioning prior to seizure onset and the epilepsy syndrome, as well as the underlying cause. In population-based studies, learning difficulties (mental handicap) are present in 21–34%, and 51–57% will be found to have some learning difficulties at the time of diagnosis of epilepsy (95).

Specific cognitive impairments have also been reported with some epilepsy syndromes. In benign epilepsy of childhood with centro-temporal spikes, a variety of neurocognitive concerns have been identified in those with active epilepsy and EEG discharges, including problems with auditory (verbal) and visuo-spatial memory, reading comprehension, visuo-motor co-ordination, picture-naming and verbal fluency and executive function (95). Several studies have correlated neurocognitive deficits with lateralization of epileptic activity. However, these deficits usually resolve with remission of seizures but, more importantly, normalization of the EEG (96, 97).

Children with remote symptomatic, partial epilepsy have a higher likelihood of pre-existing cognitive problems owing to preceding brain injury or underlying brain malformations. In addition, the seizure focus may help to predict cognitive deficits. The frontal lobe is important in sustaining attention and regulation of affect, and executive function. Predictably, children with frontal lobe epilepsy have greater problems with attention, hyperactivity, impulsivity, impaired inhibition and working memory (98). The temporal lobe has important functions in memory and receptive language. Intellectual dysfunction affects over half of patients with unilateral temporal lobe epilepsy and these children also frequently have memory impairment (99) and executive dysfunction (100), which may deteriorate with time, particularly where the pathology is mesial temporal sclerosis.

Cognitive outcome is also impaired in a significant minority of children with typical absence epilepsy. In a population-based study, 36% failed to graduate from high school, and 48% repeated at least one grade (101). Attention is often adversely affected in children with idiopathic generalized epilepsy, particularly in those with absence seizures. While frequent bursts of spike and slow wave activity correlate with greater impairment, attention deficits in absence epilepsy are not solely explained by these discharges. Antiepileptic medication, specifically with valproic acid (sodium valproate) may also contribute to some of the attention deficit.

Children with symptomatic generalized epilepsy may show developmental delay prior to the onset of seizures, and further impairment may occur, possibly because of very frequent seizures and recurrent episodes of non-convulsive status epilepticus (102); excessive polypharmacy (numbers of drugs or high doses, or both) may also contribute to any impairment. In Lennox–Gastaut syndrome, 54% were shown to have an IQ < 25. Children with myoclonic–astatic epilepsy usually demonstrate normal cognition prior to epilepsy onset but their long-term cognitive outcome is more variable and depends on seizure control, being poorer in those with ongoing tonic seizures or recurrent, non-convulsive status epilepticus. On follow-up after a mean period of over 10 years, 59% of children with myoclonic–astatic epilepsy had a normal IQ, 20% were borderline or mildly mentally handicapped, and 21% had moderate to severe mental handicap (learning difficulties) (103). Outcome is also impaired in ESESS. Normal language and intelligence is seen in only 10–44% of children long term; the longer the duration of ESESS, the poorer the outcome (103).

Social

Long-term social outcome may also be impaired in pediatric epilepsy, with lower rates of graduation from high school or further training, higher rates of unemployment or under-employment, lower marriage rates, fewer social relationships, less financial independence and lower rates of independent living (105–107). However, these outcomes may be determined primarily by the specific epilepsy syndrome and seizure control within the syndrome as well as the underlying cause of the epilepsy. Additional factors are also likely to be important, including the patient's self-esteem and adjustment to having epilepsy, as well as genetically determined personality traits.

Benign childhood epilepsy with centro-temporal spikes appears to be truly benign, with an excellent long-term social outcome. In a study of 79 patients followed for more than 15 years, social adaptability was excellent (108). Conversely, the outcome for children with symptomatic or cryptogenic focal (partial) epilepsy is often poor, particularly among those with cognitive or neurological disabilities (105, 107). Children with typical absence epilepsy may also experience difficulties. Follow-up of a population-derived cohort in early adulthood showed that they had greater academic problems, poorer occupational status, more behavior and substance abuse problems, higher rates of unplanned pregnancy and greater psychiatric morbidity than controls with non-neurological chronic disease (101). However, it must be appreciated that cultural factors may influence these findings. Finally, and predictably, the social development and outcome of those with symptomatic generalized epilepsy is poor or very poor, given the frequency of their seizures and associated cognitive impairment. One study showed that only 13% were able to live independently while 58% were dependent for nearly all activities (109). Ninety percent were completely dependent on their parents or the state and only 13% had 'significant' social interaction in community activities.

REFERENCES

1. Stephenson J, Whitehouse WP, Zuberi S. Paroxysmal nonepileptic disorders: differential diagnosis of epilepsy. In: Wallace SJ, Farrell K, eds. *Epilepsy in Children* 2nd edn. London, Arnold. 2004; 4–20.
2. Eldridge PR, Punt JA. Risks associated with giving benzodiazepines to patients with acute neurological injuries. *BMJ* 1990; **300**: 1189–90.
3. American Academy of Pediatrics: The neurodiagnostic evaluation of the child with a first simple febrile seizure. *Pediatrics* 1996; **97**: 769–72.
4. Allen JE, Ferrie CD, Livingston JH, Feltbower RG. Recovery of consciousness after epileptic seizures in children. *Arch Dis Child* 2007; **92**: 39–42.
5. Lempert T, Bauer M, Schmidt D. Syncope: a videometric analysis of 56 episodes of transient cerebral hypoxia. *Ann Neurol* 1994; **36**: 233–7.
6. Horrocks IA, Nechay A, Stephenson JB, Zuberi SM. Anoxic–epileptic seizures: observational study of epileptic seizures induced by syncopes. *Arch Dis Child* 2005; **90**: 1283–7.
7. Revised terminology and concepts for organization of the epilepsies: Report of the Commission on Classification and Terminology 2009: www.ilae-epilepsy.org/Visitors/Centre/ctf/ctfoverview.cfm.
8. Panayiotopoulos CP. Typical absence seizures and related epileptic syndromes: assessment of current state and directions for future research. *Epilepsia* 2008; **49**: 2131–9.
9. Marini C, Harkin LA, Wallace RH, *et al.* Childhood absence epilepsy and febrile seizures: a family with a GABA(A) receptor mutation. *Brain* 2003; **126**: 230–40.
10. Lillywhite LM, Saling MM, Harvey AS, *et al.* Neuropsychological and functional MRI studies provide converging evidence of anterior language dysfunction in BECTS. *Epilepsia* 2009; **50**: 2276–84.
11. Ferrie C, Caraballo R, Covanis A, *et al.* Panayiotopoulos syndrome: a consensus view. *Dev Med Child Neurol* 2006; **48**: 236–40.
12. Caraballo R, Cers'osimo R, Fejerman N. Panayiotopoulos syndrome: a prospective study of 192 patients. *Epilepsia* 2007; **48**: 1054–61.
13. Guerrini R, Parmeggiani L, Bonanni P, *et al.* Myoclonic astatic epilepsy. In: Roger J, Bureau M, Dravet C, *et al.*, eds. *Epileptic Syndromes in Infancy, Childhood and Adolescence*. Paris, John Libbey 2005; 115–24.
14. Livingston JH. Management of epilepsies associated with specific diseases in children. In: Shorvon S, Perucca E, Engel J, eds. *The Treatment of Epilepsy* 3rd edn. Oxford, Wiley–Blackwell 2009; 195–202.
15. Gaillard WD, Chiron C, Cross JH, *et al.* Guidelines for imaging infants and children with recent-onset epilepsy. *Epilepsia* 2009; **50**: 2147–53.
16. Cramer JA, Glassman M, Rienzi V. The relationship between poor medication compliance and seizures. *Epilepsy Behav* 2002; **3**: 338–42.
17. Dudley RW, Penney SJ, Buckley DJ. First-drug treatment failures in children newly diagnosed with epilepsy. *Pediatr Neurol* 2009; **40**: 71–7.
18. Carpay HA, *et al.* Epilepsy in childhood: an audit of clinical practice. *Arch Neurol* 1998; **55**: 668–73.
19. Camfield CS, Camfield PR, Veugelers PJ. Death in children with epilepsy: a population-based study. *Lancet* 2002; **359**: 1891–5.

20. Sillanpaa M, *et al.* Long-term prognosis of seizures with onset in childhood. *N Engl J Med* 1998; **338**: 1715–22.

21. Berg AT, *et al.* Mortality in childhood-onset epilepsy. *Arch Pediatr Adolesc Med* 2004; **158**: 1147–52.

22. Callenbach PM, *et al.* Mortality risk in children with epilepsy: the Dutch study of epilepsy in childhood. *Pediatrics* 2001; **107**: 1259–63.

23. Diekema DS, Quan L, Holt VL. Epilepsy as a risk factor for submersion injury in children. *Pediatrics* 1993; **91**: 612–6.

24. Kemp AM, Sibert JR. Epilepsy in children and the risk of drowning. *Arch Dis Child* 1993; **68**: 684–5.

25. Deekollu D, Besag FM, Aylett SE. Seizure-related injuries in a group of young people with epilepsy wearing protective helmets: incidence, types and circumstances. *Seizure* 2005; **14**: 347–53.

26. Samaniego EA, Sheth RD. Bone consequences of epilepsy and antiepileptic medications. *Semin Pediatr Neurol* 2007; **14**: 196–200.

27. Wirrell EC, *et al.* Accidental injury is a serious risk in children with typical absence epilepsy. *Arch Neurol* 1996; **53**: 929–32.

28. Appleton RE. The Mersey Region Pediatric Epilepsy Interest Group. Seizure-related injuries in children with newly diagnosed and untreated epilepsy. *Epilepsia* 2002; **43**: 764–7.

29. Carpay HA, *et al.* Disability due to restrictions in childhood epilepsy. *Dev Med Child Neurol* 1997; **39**: 521–6.

30. Wirrell EC, *et al.* Long-term psychosocial outcome in typical absence epilepsy. Sometimes a wolf in sheep's clothing. *Arch Pediatr Adolesc Med* 1997; **151**: 152–8.

31. Camfield C, *et al.* Biologic factors as predictors of social outcome of epilepsy in intellectually normal children: a population-based study. *J Pediatr* 1993; **122**: 869–73.

32. Jalava M, *et al.* Social adjustment and competence 35 years after onset of childhood epilepsy: a prospective controlled study. *Epilepsia* 1997; **38**: 708–15.

33. Sillanpaa M. Epilepsy in children: prevalence, disability, and handicap. *Epilepsia* 1992; **33**: 444–9.

34. Nolan MA, *et al.* Intelligence in childhood epilepsy syndromes. *Epilepsy Res* 2003; **53**: 139–50.

35. Hermann BP, *et al.* Cognitive and magnetic resonance volumetric abnormalities in new-onset pediatric epilepsy. *Semin Pediatr Neurol* 2007; **14**: 173–80.

36. Seidenberg M, Pulsipher DT, Hermann B. Cognitive progression in epilepsy. *Neuropsychol Rev* 2007; **17**: 445–54.

37. Hermann BP, *et al.* Growing up with epilepsy: A two-year investigation of cognitive development in children with new onset epilepsy. *Epilepsia* 2008; **49**: 1847–58.

38. Dunn DW, *et al.* ADHD and epilepsy in childhood. *Dev Med Child Neurol* 2003; **45**: 50–4.

39. Hermann B, *et al.* The frequency, complications and etiology of ADHD in new onset pediatric epilepsy. *Brain* 2007; **130**: 3135–48.

40. Austin JK, *et al.* Behavior problems in children before first recognized seizures. *Pediatrics* 2001; **107**: 115–22.

41. Austin JK, Dunn DW. Progressive behavioral changes in children with epilepsy. *Prog Brain Res* 2002; **135**: 419–27.

42. Sherman EM, *et al.* ADHD, neurological correlates and health-related quality of life in severe pediatric epilepsy. *Epilepsia* 2007; **48**: 1083–91.

43. Baptista-Neto L, *et al.* An expert opinion on methylphenidate treatment for attention deficit hyperactivity disorder in pediatric patients with epilepsy. *Expert Opin Investig Drugs* 2008; **17**: 77–84.
44. Rutter M, Yule GPW. *A neuropsychiatric study in childhood.* Philadelphia, Lippincott 1970.
45. Jones JE, *et al.* Psychiatric comorbidity in children with new onset epilepsy. *Dev Med Child Neurol* 2007; **49**: 493–7.
46. Ettinger AB, *et al.* Symptoms of depression and anxiety in pediatric epilepsy patients. *Epilepsia* 1998; **39**: 595–9.
47. Jones JE, *et al.* Psychiatric disorders in children and adolescents who have epilepsy. *Pediatr Rev* 2008; **29**: e9–14.
48. Wirrell E, *et al.* Sleep disturbances in children with epilepsy compared with their nearest-aged siblings. *Dev Med Child Neurol* 2005; **47**: 754–9.
49. Stores G, Wiggs L, Campling G. Sleep disorders and their relationship to psychological disturbance in children with epilepsy. *Child Care Health Dev* 1998; **24**: 5–19.
50. Koh S, *et al.* Sleep apnea treatment improves seizure-control in children with neurodevelopmental disorders. *Pediatr Neurol* 2000; **22**: 36–9.
51. Ghazziuddin M. Seizure disorder in autism spectrum disorders: an overview. In: Riva D, Rapin I, eds. *Autistic Spectrum Disorders.* Montrouge, John Libbey Eurotext 2005; 69–74.
52. Camfield PR, *et al.* If a first antiepileptic drug fails to control a child's epilepsy, what are the chances of success with the next drug? *J Pediatr* 1997; **131**: 821–4.
53. Dudley RW, Penny SJ, Buckley DJ. First-drug treatment failures in children newly diagnosed with epilepsy. *Pediatr Neurol* 2009; **40**: 71–7.
54. Uldall P, *et al.* The misdiagnosis of epilepsy in children admitted to a tertiary epilepsy centre with paroxysmal events. *Arch Dis Child* 2006; **91**: 219–21.
55. Snead OC, 3rd, Hosey LC. Exacerbation of seizures in children by carbamazepine. *N Engl J Med* 1985; **313**: 916–21.
56. Talwar D, Arora MS, Sher PK. EEG changes and seizure exacerbation in young children treated with carbamazepine. *Epilepsia* 1994; **35**: 1154–9.
57. Kochen S, Giagante B, Oddo S. Spike-and-wave complexes and seizure exacerbation caused by carbamazepine. *Eur J Neurol* 2002; **9**: 41–7.
58. Corda D, *et al.* Incidence of drug-induced aggravation in benign epilepsy with centrotemporal spikes. *Epilepsia* 2001; **42**: 754–9.
59. Lortie A, *et al.* The potential for increasing seizure frequency, relapse, and appearance of new seizure types with vigabatrin. *Neurology* 1993; **43**(Suppl 5): S24–7.
60. Tassinari CA, *et al.* Tonic status epilepticus precipitated by intravenous benzodiazepine in five patients with Lennox-Gastaut syndrome. *Epilepsia* 1972; **13**: 421–35.
61. Wheless JW, *et al.* Treatment of pediatric epilepsy: European expert opinion, 2007. *Epileptic Disord* 2007; **9**: 353–412.
62. Wheless JW, Clarke DF, Carpenter D. Treatment of pediatric epilepsy: expert opinion, 2005. *J Child Neurol* 2005; **20**(Suppl 1): S1–56; quiz S59–60.
63. Glauser TA, Cnaan A, Shinnar S, *et al.* Ethosuximide, valproic acid and lamotrigine in childhood absence epilepsy. *New Eng J Med* 2010; **362**: 790–9.
64. Glauser T, Kluger G, Sachdeo R, Krauss G, Perdorno C, Arroyo S. Rufinamide for generalized seizures associated with Lennox-Gastaut syndrome. *Neurology* 2008; **70**: 1950–8.
65. Hancock E, Cross H. Treatment of Lennox-Gastaut syndrome. *Cochrane Database Syst Rev* 2003; **3**: CD003277.
66. Neal EG, Chaffe H, Schwartz RH, *et al.* The ketogenic diet for the treatment of childhood epilepsy: a randomised controlled trial. *Lancet Neurology* 2008; **122**: 334–40.

67. Freeman JM, Vining EP, Kossoff EH, Pyzik PL, Ye X, Goodman SN. A blinded, crossover study of the efficacy of the ketogenic diet. *Epilepsia* 2009; **50**: 322–5.

68. Rating D, Wolf C, Bast T. Sulthiame as monotherapy in children with benign childhood epilepsy with centrotemporal spikes: a 6-month randomized, double-blind, placebo-controlled study. Sulthiame Study Group. *Epilepsia* 2000; **41**: 1284–8.

69. Sirven JI, Sperling M, Wingerchuk DM. Early versus late antiepileptic drug withdrawal for people with epilepsy in remission. *Cochrane Database Syst Rev* 2001; **3**: CD001902.

70. Peters AC, et al. Randomized prospective study of early discontinuation of antiepileptic drugs in children with epilepsy. *Neurology* 1998; **50**: 724–30.

71. Bouma PA, et al. The course of benign partial epilepsy of childhood with centrotemporal spikes: a meta-analysis. *Neurology* 1997; **48**: 430–7.

72. Camfield P, Camfield C. The frequency of intractable seizures after stopping AEDs in seizure-free children with epilepsy. *Neurology* 2005; **64**: 973–5.

73. Ranganathan LN, Ramaratnam S. Rapid versus slow withdrawal of antiepileptic drugs. *Cochrane Database Syst Rev* 2006; **2**: CD005003.

74. Berg AT, et al. Early development of intractable epilepsy in children: a prospective study. *Neurology* 2001; **56**: 1445–52.

75. Carpay HA, et al. Epilepsy in childhood: an audit of clinical practice. *Arch Neurol* 1998; **55**: 668–73.

76. Elkis LC, et al. Efficacy of second antiepileptic drug after failure of one drug in children with partial epilepsy. *Epilepsia* 1993; **34**(Suppl 6): 107 (Abstract).

77. Aso K, Watanabe K. Limitations in the medical treatment of cryptogenic or symptomatic localization-related epilepsies of childhood onset. *Epilepsia* 2000; **41**(Suppl 9): 18–20.

78. Spencer S, Huh L. Outcomes of epilepsy surgery in adults and children. *Lancet Neurol* 2008; **7**: 525–37.

79. Murphy JV. Left vagal nerve stimulation in children with medically refractory epilepsy. The Pediatric VNS Study Group. *J Pediatr* 1999; **134**: 563–6.

80. Buoni S, et al. Vagus nerve stimulation for drug resistant epilepsy in children and young adults. *Brain Dev* 2004; **26**: 158–63.

81. Benifla M, et al. Vagal nerve stimulation for refractory epilepsy in children: indications and experience at The Hospital for Sick Children. *Childs Nerv Syst* 2006; **22**: 1018–26.

82. Parker AP, et al. Vagal nerve stimulation in epileptic encephalopathies. *Pediatrics* 1999; **103**: 778–82.

83. Kossoff EH, et al. Optimal clinical management of children receiving the ketogenic diet: recommendations of the International Ketogenic Diet Study Group. *Epilepsia* 2009; **50**: 304–17.

84. Neal EG, et al. The ketogenic diet for the treatment of childhood epilepsy: a randomised controlled trial. *Lancet Neurol* 2008; **7**: 500–6.

85. Snead OC, 3rd, Benton JW, Myers GJ. ACTH and prednisone in childhood seizure disorders. *Neurology* 1983; **33**: 966–70.

86. Gupta R, Appleton R. Corticosteroids in the management of the paediatric epilepsies. *Arch Dis Child* 2005; **90**: 379–84.

87. Tsuru T, et al. Effects of high-dose intravenous corticosteroid therapy in Landau–Kleffner syndrome. *Pediatr Neurol* 2000; **22**: 145–7.

88. Hart YM, *et al.* Medical treatment of Rasmussen's syndrome (chronic encephalitis and epilepsy): effect of high-dose steroids or immunoglobulins in 19 patients. *Neurology* 1994; **44**: 1030–6.

89. Mikati MA, *et al.* Efficacy of intravenous immunoglobulin in Landau–Kleffner syndrome. *Pediatr Neurol* 2002; **26**: 298–300.

90. Illum N, *et al.* Intravenous immunoglobulin: a single-blind trial in children with Lennox-Gastaut syndrome. *Neuropediatrics* 1990; **21**: 87–90.

91. Camfield C, *et al.* Outcome of childhood epilepsy: a population-based study with a simple predictive scoring system for those treated with medication. *J Pediatr* 1993; **122**: 861–8.

92. Sillanpaa M, Camfield P, Camfield C. Predicting long-term outcome of childhood epilepsy in Nova Scotia, Canada, and Turku, Finland. Validation of a simple scoring system. *Arch Neurol* 1995; **52**: 589–92.

93. Wirrell EC, *et al.* Long-term prognosis of typical childhood absence epilepsy: remission or progression to juvenile myoclonic epilepsy. *Neurology* 1996; **47**: 912–8.

94. Camfield P, Camfield C. Long-term prognosis for symptomatic (secondarily) generalized epilepsies: a population-based study. *Epilepsia* 2007; **48**: 1128–32.

95. Camfield CS, Camfield PR. Long-term social outcomes for children with epilepsy. *Epilepsia* 2007; **48**(Suppl 9): 3–5.

96. Baglietto MG, *et al.* Neuropsychological disorders related to interictal epileptic discharges during sleep in benign epilepsy of childhood with centrotemporal or Rolandic spikes. *Dev Med Child Neurol* 2001; **43**: 407–12.

97. Deonna T, *et al.* Benign partial epilepsy of childhood: a longitudinal neuropsychological and EEG study of cognitive function. *Dev Med Child Neurol* 2000; **42**: 595–603.

98. Hernandez MT, *et al.* Attention, memory, and behavioral adjustment in children with frontal lobe epilepsy. *Epilepsy Behav* 2003; **4**: 522–36.

99. Gonzalez LM, *et al.* The localization and lateralization of memory deficits in children with temporal lobe epilepsy. *Epilepsia* 2007; **48**: 124–32.

100. Rzezak P, *et al.* Frontal lobe dysfunction in children with temporal lobe epilepsy. *Pediatr Neurol* 2007; **37**: 176–85.

101. Wirrell EC, *et al.* Long-term psychosocial outcome in typical absence epilepsy. Sometimes a wolf in sheep's clothing. *Arch Pediatr Adolesc Med* 1997; **151**: 152–8.

102. Berg AT, *et al.* Longitudinal assessment of adaptive behavior in infants and young children with newly diagnosed epilepsy: influences of etiology, syndrome, and seizure-control. *Pediatrics* 2004; **114**: 645–50.

103. Oguni H, *et al.* Treatment and long-term prognosis of myoclonic-astatic epilepsy of early childhood. *Neuropediatrics* 2002; **33**: 122–32.

104. Nickels K, Wirrell E. Electrical status epilepticus in sleep. *Semin Pediatr Neurol* 2008; **15**: 50–60.

105. Kokkonen J, *et al.* Psychosocial outcome of young adults with epilepsy in childhood. *J Neurol Neurosurg Psychiatry* 1997; **62**: 265–8.

106. Jalava M, *et al.* Social adjustment and competence 35 years after onset of childhood epilepsy: a prospective controlled study. *Epilepsia* 1997; **38**: 708–15.

107. Camfield C, *et al.* Biologic factors as predictors of social outcome of epilepsy in intellectually normal children: a population-based study. *J Pediatr* 1993; **122**: 869–73.

108. Loiseau P, *et al*. Long-term prognosis in two forms of childhood epilepsy: typical absence seizures and epilepsy with rolandic (centrotemporal) EEG foci. *Ann Neurol* 1983; **13**: 642–8.

109. Camfield C, Camfield P. Twenty years after childhood-onset symptomatic generalized epilepsy the social outcome is usually dependency or death: a population-based study. *Dev Med Child Neurol* 2008; **50**: 859–63.

4

Epilepsy beginning in adolescence

Tim Martland and Carol Camfield

Incidence of epilepsy during puberty and adolescence

Normal puberty begins between the ages eight and 12 years in girls and nine and 14 years in boys. The five Tanner stages of puberty are recognized as a sequence of events which occur over several years leading a child into young adulthood. It is characterized by hormonal secretions, growth spurts, development of secondary sexual characteristics and reproductive functions and behavioral changes. A common belief exists that the onset of unprovoked seizures are precipitated or caused by the initiation of puberty. However, several well-conducted epidemiological studies now refute this belief and have shown that the incidence of epilepsy is not influenced by the onset of puberty (1). This is illustrated by the population-based study of childhood epilepsy in Nova Scotia where 692 children (aged one month to 16 years) were identified at the onset of their epilepsy (1). Figure 4.1 demonstrates a decrease in the incidence of epilepsy during the years of puberty from approximately 40/100,000 under the age of nine years to 20/100,000 in older children.

Another retrospective, questionnaire-based method was undertaken in 265 Austrian women with epilepsy which focused on reproductive health issues and epilepsy (2). No significant differences were found in the age of the onset of epilepsy during the perimenarche period (two years before or after the year of menarche) compared to the five-year periods before and after perimenarche. Finally, the age at which menarche occurred did not appear to be related to the onset of epilepsy.

However, some epilepsy syndromes are influenced by gender and show an age of onset that does appear to coincide with puberty. For example, juvenile absence epilepsy (JAE) is more frequent in females with an onset at or older than 10 years of age. Similarly, two-thirds of those who have juvenile myoclonic epilepsy (JME) are women and the syndrome usually develops during adolescence, with a peak age of ten

Childhood Epilepsy: Management from Diagnosis to Remission, ed. Richard Appleton and Peter Camfield. Published by Cambridge University Press. © Cambridge University Press 2011.

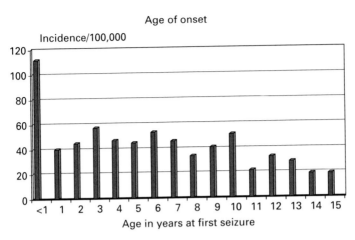

Figure 4.1 Incidence of epilepsy by age at onset.

to 16 years, although with a considerably wider age range (eight to 24 years). In comparison, it is interesting that benign epilepsy with centro-temporal spikes (BECTS or benign rolandic epilepsy of childhood [BREC]) always ends by mid-adolescence. For these disorders it is not clear if puberty itself has an influence or if the timing of onset or remission is related to age or some other, and specific, genetically determined factor. Finally, it is interesting to note that terminal remission after discontinuation of antiepileptic drugs (AEDs) after a one, two, three, four or five-year period of seizure freedom is unrelated to the age or time since the onset of puberty.

Effects of puberty on established epilepsy

Hippocrates was the first to suggest a possible association between puberty and epilepsy, noting a more benign course during puberty and that seizures often could either reduce in intensity or even remit during this period. Over 2,000 years later, there is very little additional information on the effect of puberty and its interaction with seizure control for children who develop epilepsy before puberty. One old and very small study followed 39 children with epilepsy from pre-puberty into puberty and noted no change in seizure control following the onset of puberty (3).

The diagnosis of epilepsy in adolescence: common problems

The diagnosis of epilepsy is generally based on a detailed and accurate history, irrespective of the person's age. The information given by the patient and their family is frequently incomplete because of the patient's partial or complete loss of consciousness during part of the episode. Therefore, a witness to the event is needed who can fill in the parts that are missing and reinforce the details given from the memory of the teenager. In addition, teenagers (adolescents) may not always

Table 4.1 Comparison between epilepsy, convulsive syncope and NEAD

Symptom	Epilepsy	Vasovagal syncope	Non-epileptic attack disorder
Provocation	Only occasional triggers (see below); most occur 'anywhere, anytime and any place'	Yes, but may not be recognized unless specifically questioned	Emotional and situational (often quite public); rarely occur when alone
Pallor	Unusual	Nearly always	Rarely
Family history of a first-degree relative	10–15%	Usually, probably an autosomal dominant gene with incomplete penetrance	Occasionally (may act as a template for episodes)
Tonic seizure	Usually seen in secondary generalized epilepsies with associated neuro-developmental delay	50% (very brief)	May be seen but unsustained (interspersed with periods of immobility) and inconsistent
Myoclonus or clonic movements	Seen with specific epilepsy syndromes	Frequent, but very brief (seconds only)	Common but less 'shock-like'
Onset	Sudden (tonic component)	Gradual	Variable; usually sudden (if the 'seizure' is a tonic-clonic seizure)
Offset	Gradual reduction in frequency of clonic movements before stopping	Sudden cessation	Sudden (if the 'seizure' is a tonic-clonic seizure)
Duration	Varies from seconds to many minutes	Generally less than 60 seconds	Often prolonged and repeated
Recurrence	50% after first seizure; 80% after second	Frequent	Frequent – even many times a day

appreciate the significance of odd sensations (which may represent auras – simple partial sensory seizures) or early morning jerks (which may represent myoclonic seizures) and fail to mention or report this information spontaneously.

Because there are many different types of seizures and epilepsy syndromes, there are many ways that the adolescent may present to the clinician. It has been reported that up to 50% of paroxysmal events, initially considered to be epileptic in origin, are caused by another paroxysmal, but non-epileptic disorder. There are a number of conditions that may cause some confusion and be misdiagnosed as epilepsy; two of the most common are syncope and non-epileptic attack disorder (Table 4.1).

Convulsive syncope

Convulsive syncope is a sudden loss of consciousness associated with the inability to maintain postural tone, usually in association with brief extensor stiffening and a few seconds of symmetric or asymmetric myoclonus. Sometimes the person may be incontinent of urine but will only very rarely bite their tongue. The person does not usually complain of any post-syncopal drowsiness and usually recovers rapidly, within ten to 20 minutes. An eye-witness account is often necessary to confirm the diagnosis and will report that the person is pale or 'deathly white.' However, it is always important to ask the teenager about how they felt around the time of the episode – as they will commonly describe clear pre-syncopal symptoms, including feeling light-headed or 'dizzy', cold and clammy, 'distant' and with altered hearing (voices sounding muffled or like an 'echo') or visual disturbances (blurry or tunnel vision) and even being aware that they are about to fall; failing to ask these questions of the teenager may miss important information.

The cause of vasovagal syncope is a sudden failure of the autonomic nervous system to maintain blood pressure and bradycardia that leads to decreased cerebral perfusion of oxygenated blood. As the hypoxia deepens, a convulsive seizure is common. As Stephenson asserts, the anoxic seizure follows because of a marked decrease or 'an abrupt cutting off of energy substrates to the cerebral cortex.' (4)

The vasovagal syncopal event has a lifetime prevalence of approximately 30% and is a relatively common event in adolescence. A population-based study from Rochester, USA found an incidence of 71–125/100,000 with a peak incidence in those aged 15–19 years. A retrospective study evaluated 443 patients (aged 18–70 years) with one or more episodes of vasovagal syncope and found the modal age for a first episode of syncope to be three years. In a smaller case series of 113 children who had attended a pediatric emergency room with a diagnosis of vasovagal syncope, the mean age at the time of the syncope was 14.8 +/− 3.3 years.

Provoking factors for convulsive syncope are well known. In a large cross-sectional study of 549 members of a general population, the more frequently cited triggers of syncope included: acute illness, warm environment, pain, insufficient food intake, seeing blood or undergoing venepuncture, or a strong emotion. The most important element in the diagnosis of syncope is the situation or context in which the event occurred, and what the adolescent was doing at that time. If the situation is one in which syncope is a common occurrence, then it is very likely to be the underlying diagnosis.

Vasovagal syncope usually has a gradual onset of premonitory symptoms as described earlier; recurrences will have similar if not identical symptoms and signs. Syncope is accompanied by hypotension and bradycardia. When consciousness is regained, weakness and 'fuzzy' or 'muddled' thinking may last a number of minutes and the loss of consciousness and myoclonic or clonic movements cannot be recalled.

For most, a clear history of the event and detailed family, dietary and past medical history, together with the physical examination, will be all that is needed for diagnosis. However, if the episodes are repeated and are not obviously associated with either clearly identified provoking factors or premonitory (pre-syncopal) symptoms, or both, or there are more epileptic-sounding features to the episodes, then a video recording of the episodes may be helpful, although this may be difficult to obtain. If the diagnosis remains in doubt and is tending more towards one of epilepsy, then a sleep-deprived EEG may be indicated.

Occasionally, this type of event in a young patient may represent a potentially life-threatening disorder, and specifically the congenital prolonged QT interval syndrome, Wolff–Parkinson-White (WPW) syndrome, Brugada syndrome, or hypertrophic cardiomyopathy. Therefore, it is essential to undertake a formal 12-lead electrocardiogram (ECG) in all children and teenagers who experience paroxysmal episodes or apparent syncope in association with exercise or a sudden startle. An ECG should also be obtained in those teenagers in whom there is a family history of sudden cardiac death. An exercise ECG should be obtained or the teenager referred for a formal cardiovascular opinion if the initial, routine ECG is normal but an underlying cardiac arrhythmia remains a distinct possibility. Finally, a full blood count should also be checked because syncope may be the presenting feature of anemia.

Non-epileptic attack disorder (NEAD); also called psychogenic non-epileptic seizures (PNES) or 'pseudo-epileptic seizures'

Non-epileptic seizures are a common clinical problem in adolescents and may cause significant diagnostic confusion, and particularly when they occur in teenagers who also have definite epileptic seizures. The clinician has to try and decide whether the reported events are caused by epilepsy or whether some, or all, may be non-epileptic seizures, previously called 'pseudo-seizures.' Seventy-five percent of adolescents with non-epileptic seizures also have epilepsy. In a quarter of patients with NEAD there may be a family history of epilepsy which may provide a model used for imitation; other 'models' frequently include a close friend who has epilepsy. The vast majority of NEAD is diagnosed in children aged 12 years and above. In a number of clinical series of children undergoing long-term video–EEG monitoring in the United States, up to 20% experienced non-epileptic seizures. It is important to remember that NEAD may also occur in children with mild or even moderate learning difficulties, as well as those with no cognitive impairment.

The main issue for the clinician faced with an adolescent with potentially non-epileptic seizures is diagnostic. Once again, it is important to obtain an accurate and detailed history of the episodes and particularly from one or more eye witnesses; video recordings may also prove helpful if not diagnostic. Often the diagnosis of NEAD is not clear until an episode is captured on video or witnessed by an experienced clinician. Some patients may be induced to have a seizure through suggestion, in the clinic. The question of whether events may be NEAD is often raised when a new seizure type develops, or there appears to be an evolution, or a worsening in severity of previous seizure types.

When non-epileptic seizures occur, most families assume that it is related to a change in their child's epilepsy and may be extremely concerned about the potential evolution of a more serious problem. It may take some considerable time to convince the family that these, often more dramatic episodes, are not epileptic in origin. It may be necessary to use techniques such as prolonged EEG or video–EEG monitoring to not only confirm the diagnosis, but also to enable the family to be confident with their child's clinician. Reviewing video footage with the family and explaining why the episodes are non-epileptic in origin is a useful therapeutic step.

If the discussion of non-epileptic seizures is not handled in a sensitive and understanding manner, the relationship between the clinician and a young person and their family can be adversely affected – and the family will frequently request a second or third opinion. In our experience, resolution of non-epileptic seizures only occurs if the family or carers and others (e.g., friends, school or college staff) who are significantly involved with the young person are convinced of, and 'buy-in' to the diagnosis of non-epileptic seizures. When doubt remains in their minds, the tendency will be to side with the young person, and assume that this is a genuine change in the epilepsy and merits further investigations and treatment. When such events happen at school, especially when prolonged, there are often significant implications for access to school services for the young person; this can include the child being suspended from school, an action justified by the school because it is in the young person's 'best interests' or because the school or college will not take responsibility for the young person. Input about epilepsy and NEAD from an epilepsy specialist nurse to educate the school staff about non-epileptic seizures and their management can be very important in assuring continued access to education and the provision of a socially appropriate situation.

It is frequently thought that NEAD is a marker for psychological or psychiatric illness, but this is rarely the case. For example, a formal psychiatric diagnosis of depression is found in less than 25% of young people with NEAD, although some psychological stresses such as difficulties at school (bullying, failing to achieve or not meeting their own expectations or those of their parents), family discord and interpersonal difficulties can often be identified by a careful, detailed – and importantly, patiently obtained – history. These are common accompaniments of adolescence and do not necessarily indicate a psychiatric or psychological disorder. In the literature, prominence is given to the association between non-epileptic seizures and child abuse, particularly sexual abuse, but in British practice this appears to be far less prominent than it would appear from the literature. In the USA by contrast, approximately one-third of young females with NEAD will be found to have to been exposed to major sexual abuse or have identity problems. A careful and gentle exploration of psychological and psychiatric issues should be undertaken but ideally this should be undertaken by specialized child and/or adolescent mental health personnel. Such services are not always available in many countries and even when they are, there may be considerable waiting times. One of the most important factors that is associated with a successful diagnosis and management (and therefore outcome), is early diagnosis: to consider the diagnosis as early as possible avoids inappropriate investigations, an escalation of antiepileptic drug treatment and the avoidance of multiple medical opinions.

It is also important that, when giving the diagnosis of NEAD, the clinician is non-confrontational, acknowledges that they realize that the episodes are genuine and that there is a reason for them, and positive that they can be treated but not with more and more medications. Generally, the long-term prognosis for young people with non-epileptic seizures is good, although they may be very persistent. This is usually when the diagnosis has been delayed for some years and earlier management approaches have been accusatory and non-supportive (5).

Common epilepsy syndromes seen during adolescence

Idiopathic generalized epilepsies

Juvenile absence epilepsy (JAE) is not discussed in detail in this chapter. It is an epilepsy syndrome with somewhat unclear characteristics and defining criteria. In particular, epileptologists cannot agree on the inclusion criteria, including age of onset or whether myoclonus must be present. However, all agree that it falls within the spectrum of idiopathic generalized epilepsy. It is also agreed that absence seizures are its predominant seizure type and that frequently, the syndrome evolves into juvenile myoclonic epilepsy (JME). Some consider that JAE should be omitted from the classification system of the International League Against Epilepsy (ILAE) but all agree that more detailed epidemiological and longitudinal studies are needed to clarify whether JAE is a specific epilepsy syndrome; this may be facilitated by the identification of one or more specific genetic mutations.

Idiopathic generalized epilepsy (IGE) otherwise unclassifable

Some older teenagers (aged > 13 years) present with two or more generalized tonic-clonic seizures and normal intelligence, have a normal neurological examination, show generalized spike and wave on EEG and a normal MRI. These are all features of an idiopathic generalized epilepsy but do not fulfill the criteria of the well-defined epilepsy syndromes. In the ensuing months other seizure types may occur which allow a more specific epilepsy syndrome diagnosis. Previously, some of these young people would have been diagnosed with 'epilepsy with grand mal on wakening,' but the seizures do not always occur at this time.

Juvenile myoclonic epilepsy (JME)

Myoclonic seizures are a mandatory seizure type to make the diagnosis of juvenile myoclonic epilepsy (JME); there should also be a history of at least one generalized tonic-clonic seizure, and over 60% of children and young people will experience at least one tonic-clonic seizure. Absence seizures frequently occur but are not necessary for the diagnosis. No other seizure types should occur, either at diagnosis or during follow-up. Two-thirds of patients are female. Neurological examination and cognitive function are usually normal, although some behavioral characteristics have been described in young people with JME. The inter-ictal EEG should demonstrate a normal background with bursts of fast generalized spike and wave activity with a frequency of ≥ 3 Hz. The spike and wave may be regular or irregular and may include polyspike and wave activity. Photosensitivity is present in at least 30%, but possibly 60 or 70%. Brain imaging with magnetic resonance imaging (MRI) is rarely, if ever, justified but if undertaken is usually normal; however, high-resolution MRI may show possible subtle focal cortical dysplasia, particularly within the frontal lobes.

Juvenile myoclonic epilepsy is a distinct idiopathic generalized epilepsy syndrome which most commonly presents in adolescence, with a peak age of 12–16 years. Although well described many years earlier by Janz, the syndrome came to be more commonly recognized following the influential paper of Delgado-Escueta and Enrile-Bacsal in 1984 (6). The definition is unambiguous, but often problems arise for the clinician when considering the diagnosis. There are many potential pitfalls and caveats:

- The age of onset is generally said to occur with the onset of adolescence, but in reality the age range in several large case series may be as early as eight years and may extend into early adulthood.
- The patient may present with a first seizure or several generalized tonic-clonic seizures and an inter-ictal EEG may show generalized spike-wave complexes, but without myoclonus until several years pass. The epilepsy syndrome would be classified initially as an unclassified IGE, until myoclonus develops or is first recognized, usually in the mid-teenage years.
- Myoclonus is hard to recognize and is rarely mentioned or acknowledged by the adolescent or family who feel that 'jerks' may be normal and part of waking up. To clarify this – for the young person and their family – it may be useful to discuss the universal experience of normal sleep myoclonus and also to demonstrate a typical jerk. Myoclonus is frequently observed during an EEG recording, particularly if the teenager is sleep-deprived and also during photic stimulation, but also in the outpatient clinic.
- Approximately 15% of children with childhood absence epilepsy (CAE) eventually develop JME (7). The CAE may or may not have been in remission before the symptoms of JME subsequently emerge.
- A difficult treatment decision often arises when the adolescent presents with a single generalized tonic-clonic (GTC) seizure. A history of myoclonus must be specifically sought from both the young person and their family. The myoclonus may have been occurring for weeks or months – but may have been ignored by everyone, or regarded as being a rather amusing phenomenon. The adolescent often discounts the myoclonus as trivial and refuses to accept it as an epileptic seizure because they want to be normal just like their peers and not start medication. If an EEG is obtained it will usually be abnormal and the natural history of JME means that one or more GTCs are highly likely to occur. The family and clinician are more concerned about safety, the stigma of additional seizures and achieving a significant duration of seizure freedom to enable the teenager to apply for a provisional driving licence. Seizure freedom has additional and potentially major beneficial consequences for both career choice and overall 'quality of life'.

• Because a history of myoclonus is hard to elicit, the EEG is considered to play a pivotal role in diagnosing JME after a first GTC seizure. An evidence-based review by the Quality Standards Subcommittee of the American Academy of Neurology in its Practice Parameter states, 'The majority of evidence from Class I and Class II studies confirms that an EEG helps in determination of seizure type, epilepsy syndrome, and risk for recurrence, and therefore may affect further management decisions. Experts commonly recommend that an EEG be performed after all first nonfebrile seizures' (8). Currently in North America and Australia an EEG appears to be more frequently obtained after a first afebrile seizure than in the United Kingdom. It is North American practice that the EEG be obtained after being sleep-deprived (but non-sedated) and obtained as soon as possible after the young person has recovered from their immediate post-ictal state. Clearly, this can only be achieved with adequate EEG resources, and this will vary from country to country, and even within a country.

The choice of antiepileptic medication for JME requires careful thought. If a history of myoclonic and/or absence seizures is not obtained or sought, carbamazepine may be prescribed. Unfortunately, carbamazepine is very likely to exacerbate myoclonic and absence seizures – as is phenytoin and vigabatrin. Valproic acid (sodium valproate) has been recommended as first-line treatment for many years and it continues to be the most effective AED for the seizures. However, there is increasing concern about this drug because of side effects during adolescence particularly weight gain, polycystic ovaries and teratogenicity, should the teenage girl become pregnant. Even in the absence of major or minor congenital anomalies, children born to young women who received sodium valproate, either as monotherapy or combination therapy during early pregnancy, may show learning difficulties and specifically communication difficulties.

Other AEDs may be effective, including levetiracetam (which has a specific licence as adjunctive treatment in young people aged > 12 years with JME), lamotrigine, clobazam, zonisamide, topiramate and, rarely, primidone. No adequately powered, randomized 'head-to-head' trials have specifically compared these drugs in JME. In the absence of good data, a clinical decision has to be made (9, 10). The best seizure control is likely with valproic acid (sodium valproate) but the fewest side effects are found with the other AEDs, other than possibly topiramate with its potential cognitive, language and appetite-suppressant effects. If the side effects are of greatest concern the preferred alternatives are levetiracetam or lamotrigine.

Most experts agree that JME has little chance of spontaneous remission and requires lifelong treatment. In contrast, most adolescents disagree and this can cause a problem. The study of Delgado-Escueta and Enrile-Bascal noted that 86% of their 43 patients had remission of their convulsions with valproic acid but 12 of the 13 who discontinued medication experienced a seizure relapse (6). Others have recently stated, 'In our experience not a single patient has been seizure-free after medication was withdrawn.' (11) In contrast, a recent population-based study of JME suggested that over 20–30 years of follow-up approximately, one-third of patients are successfully able to discontinue AED treatment (12).

From the adolescent's point of view, a lifetime of treatment is neither comprehensible nor sensible; it is also not perceived as a relevant option at the time of diagnosis. They will require proof that the seizures will not spontaneously remit. On the other hand, recurrent unpredictable generalized seizures are also incompatible with a teenager's expected or hoped-for lifestyle, self-esteem, confidence and peer acceptance. Treatment for a couple of years may be an acceptable alternative with subsequent discontinuation of AED treatment, clearly taking the risk that a recurrence will not happen. The timing of drug discontinuation should be tailored to the individual and their circumstances; it would be unwise and inappropriate to withdraw an AED prior to important school or college examinations, foreign travel or an imminent application for a driving licence.

Management practices for JME vary widely within both North America and Europe, including daily AED treatment for many years, short-term treatment for one to two years or no initial treatment. When JME is diagnosed after a first GTC seizure, we often decide with the family to wait for a second GTC before treatment. If two or certainly three GTC have occurred prior to the diagnosis, medication is recommended; even then, some are very hesitant and may prefer to wait for further seizures. Knowledge that even a myoclonic seizure may prevent them applying for a driving licence may be a strong motivator for many (but not all) young people to consider early treatment with an AED. In the interim, first aid for recurrent seizures is reviewed, internet websites are offered for education (i.e., www.epilepsy.com, Epilepsy Foundation of America or Epilepsy Action) and the family is provided with an individualized management plan should a recurrence occur.

Focal epilepsy: general themes

Epilepsies in which the seizures have a focal onset are the most frequent type of epilepsy seen in adolescents. It is important to identify through a very detailed history, physical examination and investigations both the origin of these seizures (generalized or focal, and the precise localization within the brain) and the epilepsy syndrome, but also the underlying cause. Many children with focal seizures also have additional specific cognitive and physical impairments. These young people often require a more detailed assessment, including psychological and psychiatric evaluations.

It is considered to be very helpful to define the child's epilepsy syndrome in order to offer correct treatment. Unfortunately, experts disagree about the syndrome classification of an individual child in at least 15%. In addition, as the child's epilepsy evolves, almost 'making itself known,' the syndrome will change in 15–20% of cases. Finally, even with the benefit of time, it may still not be possible to classify a child's (including a teenager's) epilepsy further than the first major category – idiopathic generalized, symptomatic generalized, idiopathic partial and symptomatic partial epilepsy. Early in the course of epilepsy, syndrome misdiagnosis may have little impact because with only a few exceptions treatment options will not be substantially different. It will be important to delineate epilepsy syndromes in which certain treatment choices may worsen the seizures. Examples include: carbamazepine and phenytoin may exacerbate the absence seizures and myoclonic seizures that occur in the generalized epilepsies; partial epilepsies do not respond to ethosuximide; Dravet's syndrome (severe myoclonic epilepsy in infancy) may be exacerbated by lamotrigine; and benign rolandic epilepsy does not respond to gabapentin. A number of specific syndromes are notoriously difficult to clearly distinguish. The importance of the distinction is not only in the choice of the first AED, but also in the prognosis – and therefore the information that is given to the young person and their family. While it is important to try and classify the epilepsy syndrome as soon as possible, it is important to keep an open mind – the original syndrome diagnosis may be incorrect or the syndrome may evolve and change over time. In addition, there may be an underlying and progressive underlying cause.

Seizures with a focal onset have symptoms related to the part of the brain where the initial onset occurs. They may be broadly classified into motor, sensory, autonomic or cognitive symptomatology. The initial features are often described as an 'aura' and actually represent a focal seizure without impairment of awareness. Understanding the different ictal symptoms and how these relate to the different lobes of the brain is extremely important for classification of the seizure type and epilepsy syndrome.

There are particular features of focal seizures which allow the expert clinician to pinpoint with some degree of accuracy the exact area of origin within the brain which give rise to the seizure. In studies of video–EEG recordings the correct lobe was identified through the history in all temporal lobe seizures and 74% of frontal lobe seizures. Lateralization is also highly accurate in this situation being correct in 82% of temporal and 87% of frontal lobe seizures. The clinical semiology of focal seizures in the adolescent age group is almost always the same as seen in adults, although in children younger than six or eight years the clinical features vary and they may also not be able to describe any auras accurately. Inpatient video–EEG telemetry may be helpful, if not diagnostic, in young people undergoing pre-surgical evaluation; this is also true for clinically confusing events as in sleep-related disorders and psychogenic non-epileptic seizures (13).

Unless the seizure can be confidently classified as being part of one of the recognized benign focal epilepsy syndromes, it is recommended by most clinicians that neuro-imaging should be undertaken (8). There is no doubt that magnetic resonance imaging (MRI) is superior to computed tomography (CT) and will usually identify the cause for most symptomatic epilepsies. Computerized tomography scanning has a much lower yield and may easily miss lesions that would benefit from surgical intervention.

Temporal lobe seizures

Seizures starting in the temporal lobe are probably the most common type of focal epilepsy that begins in adolescence. The majority of temporal lobe seizures begin with an 'aura' – a very short focal sensory, autonomic or motor seizure without impairment of awareness. The most common aura is an unpleasant epigastric sensation which is often described as a feeling that the stomach is rising, rolling, or fluttering. Other patients may experience a feeling of fear or panic, or describe that their thinking is disordered or memory is affected. Sensations of déjà vu or jamais vu are common. Most patients have the same aura every time. After several seconds the seizure may then cease (classified as a simple partial seizure) or it may spread with the development of additional ictal features. This may include impairment of awareness, motor arrest, bizarre behavior and automatisms (classified as a complex partial seizure) which may also terminate, or spread ('generalize') and involve the contralateral lobe with generalized convulsive movements and complete loss of consciousness; this is classified as a secondary generalized seizure.

Ninety per cent of patients with seizures from the temporal lobe will experience both an aura and loss of awareness as the seizure progresses. It is often only at this point that the seizure becomes apparent to an observer. There may be motor arrest and staring, often associated with facial pallor that may last for up to a minute. Automatisms including simple gestures or repetitive/purposeless movements often involving the oral and facial muscles and extremities are commonly seen both during the seizure and as a post-ictal phenomenon; there may be eye or head deviation to one side, or both. Nose-rubbing is a particularly common post-ictal automatism. When the dominant temporal lobe is involved speech arrest or dis-ordered language is common; however, this may also be a feature of focal seizures arising from the dominant frontal lobe. Autonomic phenomena including pallor, salivation, tachycardia and nausea can accompany temporal lobe seizures. The seizure may then progress to a secondary generalized tonic-clonic convulsion. The length of time from the onset of the aura to the completion of the seizure is usually only two or three minutes but post-ictal confusion may last for hours and the person may also sleep.

Temporal lobe seizures most commonly arise from the medial temporal lobe structures. When they arise from the lateral temporal lobe, there are often more prominent focal motor, visual or auditory symptoms. Secondary generalization that results in a tonic-clonic convulsion is seen much more frequently in lateral temporal lobe seizures.

The routine inter-ictal EEG in medial temporal lobe epilepsy is normal in two-thirds of patients. One-third will show an 'epileptic discharge' (sharp or spike and slow-wave discharges) over the anterior temporal leads, especially if the EEG includes sleep or is a prolonged recording. If an actual seizure is recorded the ictal patterns are distinctive although variable. If only an aura is recorded there will be no change on EEG. It is interesting that EEG changes may precede the clinical seizure onset by up to 30 seconds and commonly comprise increasing rhythmical activity in the theta range or low-amplitude fast (beta) activity over the temporal leads. On other occasions the patient may have significant symptoms for many seconds before there is any change on the scalp EEG.

Magnetic resonance imaging is very important in patients with temporal lobe seizures. In some neurosurgical series, abnormalities have been reported in up to 90% of patients. There are different techniques for MR scanning and a report of a 'normal' scan should not prevent referral to a specialist centre for further imaging and investigations. Although rarely available even in tertiary medical centres, high-resolution (3.0 T) MR scanning, functional imaging using PET scans and SPECT scans or magnetic resonance spectroscopy (MRS) can sometimes reveal abnormalities in the medial temporal lobe (or other focal areas from which epileptic discharges may arise) that are not visible on routine MR brain sequences.

Frontal lobe epilepsy

This is the second most common lobe for focal seizures during adolescence. The frontal lobe comprises almost 40% of the brain by volume. With seizure onset possible across such a wide area it is not surprising that the clinical and EEG manifestations of frontal lobe epilepsy vary widely and exact localization within the frontal lobe can be very difficult. Even lateralization (to one or other lobe) may not be clear. Frontal lobe seizures are of particular importance because they are frequently misdiagnosed as non-epileptic seizures or a parasomnia (specifically, night terrors) and are often resistant to anticonvulsant therapy.

The features of frontal lobe epilepsy are predominantly motor and auras are uncommon. Seizure onset in the motor cortex often presents with clonic jerks, which can be in the hand or face with spread to the arm or leg. There may also be facial distortion or speech impairment or even arrest. Loud vocalizations are quite common. Seizures that begin in the supplementary motor cortex often show very complex motor automatisms with bilateral, often asymmetrical, tonic posturing and sometimes bizarre hyperkinetic movements (e.g., repeated cycling, leg abduction or pelvic thrusting) which to an observer (and some inexperienced clinicians), can appear to be voluntary. Auras, if they occur, are usually manifest by an abnormal somatic sensation. Consciousness may be preserved, even during a frontal lobe seizure with bilateral motor involvement and this may lead to the seizure being considered to be a non-epileptic event.

There are some characteristics of frontal lobe seizures which can be very helpful in the history, including:
- the seizures tend to have a very abrupt onset and offset
- are brief
- are frequent and may occur many times a night
- predominantly, and occasionally may only, occur from sleep
- post-ictal recovery is often very quick with no confusion
- the person will return to sleep almost immediately.

Because temporal lobe seizures are common and may have a rapid spread to the frontal lobe (owing to the abundant connecting pathways between the two lobes), it is important to be able to differentiate between the two seizure types. (Table 4.2)

It can also be difficult to differentiate frontal lobe seizures from sleep disorders such as night terrors, particularly if the EEG shows no significant change during the episodes, or shows only movement artifact. Factors which make it more likely that events are frontal lobe seizures include the frequency and occasional secondary generalized tonic-clonic seizures. If more than two episodes occur per night and if the events are very stereotyped over many months, they are more likely to be

Table 4.2 Semiological features in temporal and frontal lobe seizures

Observed features	Temporal lobe	Frontal lobe
Time of seizure	Any time	Nocturnal predominance
Onset	Gradual	Abrupt
Seizure progression	Slow	Rapid
Quiet stare	Common	Unusual
Aura	Common: abdominal, sensory, autonomic or cognitive	Rare: somatosensory
Motor features	Usually subtle	Prominent (hyperkinetic; dystonic)
Automatisms	Oro-motor	Bipedal; hyperkinetic; cycling
Seizure duration	2 or 3+ minutes	30–60 seconds
Post-ictal confusion	Present for minutes	Absent or very brief
Temporal pattern	Occasional, scattered	Tend to cluster
Diurnal pattern	During wakefulness	From sleep

seizures. It is important during assessment to consider the differential diagnosis of motor movements including the paroxysmal and involuntary movement disorders or a non-epileptic event (NEAD or psychogenic non-epileptic seizures). Psychogenic non-epileptic seizures do not arise from sleep and are typically longer than the minute or two of frontal seizures; however, wild thrashing with vocalization or shouting during a frontal lobe seizure (the 'hyperkinetic' type of frontal seizure), may be so bizarre that NEAD may be the initial diagnosis, including a possible manifestation of sexual abuse. This emphasizes the importance of seeking specialist pediatric epilepsy advice. It is frequently necessary to obtain one or more video recordings of the episodes – not only at home but also in hospital using video–EEG telemetry.

Frontal lobe epilepsy, although more commonly resistant to antiepileptic medication, may still be associated with long periods of remission. However, long-term seizure control (including seizure freedom) is usually only possible with surgery (in 50–60%).

Progressive myoclonic epilepsy (PME)

One of the diagnostic difficulties that can arise in adolescents with epilepsy is distinguishing a relatively benign epilepsy syndrome from a progressive disorder. An important alarm bell or 'red flag' is when a young person presents with a prominent myoclonic element to their seizures. Young people who are later diagnosed as having a progressive myoclonic epilepsy (PME) may present with very similar symptoms to children with juvenile myoclonic epilepsy or another idiopathic generalized epilepsy.

One of the clinical clues which can help distinguish these conditions is the nature of the myoclonus. In JME the myoclonus is typically in the morning soon after waking and is subtle or minor in degree and also brief and fragmentary. In a progressive myoclonic epilepsy the myoclonus may be spread throughout the day and be marked, if not dramatic. Often it has the characteristics of action myoclonus triggered by use of a limb and is frequently stimulus-sensitive, particularly in response to touch or noise. The EEG of young people with PME often shows marked photosensitivity. Although this can be seen in JME, it is much more prominent. In PME photic stimulation may trigger myoclonus. There is no single distinguishing feature which can allow the clinician to differentiate between an idiopathic generalized epilepsy and PME at the time of presentation. Progressive myoclonic epilepsy is very rare but devastating. Awareness of the differential diagnosis and keeping an open mind if the young person's epilepsy deteriorates is important. It is particularly important not to automatically ascribe any deterioration to the teenager having an 'atypical' form of JME or poor compliance with medication. A repeat EEG may subsequently show more frequent polyspike and wave activity but also an increasingly diffusely slow background, a feature not seen in JME.

There are two main types of PME that begin during adolescence. Unverricht–Lundborg disease (ULD) is the more common form and is an autosomal recessive condition which has an onset between the ages of eight and 16 years (very similar to JME). It is caused by a mutation in the cystatin B gene (EPM1 gene). The predominant clinical features are stimulus-sensitive myoclonus, occasional generalized tonic-clonic seizures, ataxia and dysarthria. The latter two symptoms may take several years to develop following the onset of epilepsy and explains why the diagnosis is often delayed. Patients with this condition, though mentally alert, often have mild learning difficulties and show a slow progressive deterioration in cognitive functioning. Emotional lability and depression are relatively common associated features. The seizures may be partly controlled with valproic acid (sodium valproate) or levetiracetam. Resistant myoclonus may be helped by clonazepam or piracetam. Other antiepileptic drugs and specifically phenytoin or carbamazepine may worsen the seizures and may even accelerate the rate of cognitive decline.

Lafora body disease (LBD) is caused by a mutation in the gene EPM2a. This gene produces a protein (laforin) which is thought to be important in regulating neuronal function. A second gene (EPM2b) has also been described which codes for another protein found on the endoplasmic reticulum (malin). This disorder is an autosomal recessive condition and usually presents between 12 and 15 years with frequent myoclonus, but tonic-clonic seizures, ataxia and progressive cognitive decline rapidly follow. The deterioration is pronounced in Lafora body disease with affected people often dying in their twenties. The myoclonus in this condition may be seen when resting or on action. Although it may respond to the same type of drugs used in ULD, it is often resistant and disabling. The diagnosis of both ULD and LBD has been greatly facilitated by the identification of specific genetic mutations.

Other potential causes of a PME include mitochondrial disease (and not just 'MERRF' – 'myoclonic epilepsy with ragged red fibres on muscle biopsy'), juvenile neuronal ceroid lipofuscinosis, dentatorubral-pallidoluysan atrophy (DRPLA), adrenoleucodystrophy and subacute sclerosing panencephalitis (SSPE). Although these rare disorders usually show additional clinical and EEG features that help to differentiate them from the idiopathic generalized epilepsies, their initial presentation may be very similar to both JAE and JME.

Principles of drug treatment in adolescents

When a young person is diagnosed as having epilepsy, this can be a particularly difficult time for not only them but also their family. This also includes the decision as to whether to start antiepileptic drug (AED) treatment. Many families perceive AEDs as potentially harmful and almost guaranteed to cause unpleasant side effects, including drowsiness, cognitive impairment and behavior problems. There are a number of general principles that must be considered when introducing an AED in this population.

The first is to have a high degree of certainty about the diagnosis of epilepsy, the seizure types, and where possible, the specific epilepsy syndrome. It is generally accepted that an AED should be started after a second epileptic seizure. Some families prefer to wait, particularly if these seizures have been separated by a long time interval or are not major (i.e., not a tonic-clonic seizure). In other adolescents, particularly because of the motivation of possessing a driver's licence, the decision may be to start treatment after a single seizure. The decision to introduce an AED may need particular careful consideration and discussion of those situations where there may be a high risk of recurrence, as in a symptomatic epilepsy syndrome or JME, or if the initial seizure was prolonged or required intensive care management. The option of treatment should be carefully considered and addressed. The fear and anxiety induced in the family by witnessing the first epileptic seizure is great but families will gain significant reassurance by careful and patient explanation of the benign nature of the majority of such dramatic events – and 50% of those who experience a first seizure will never have another seizure.

A number of national guidelines and practice parameters have been produced to help guide and even direct clinicians in their choice of drug treatment as well as the overall care of children with epilepsy. In the UK guidelines produced by the National Institute for Health and Clinical Excellence (NICE) and the Scottish Intercollegiate Guidelines Network (SIGN) are comprehensive and based on either existing clinical evidence (14, 15) or what is regarded as 'good clinical practice' (GCP). Similar evidence-based practice parameters also exist in North America which address in detail the evaluation of a first non-febrile seizure (8) and the treatment of a child with a first unprovoked seizure (16).

These guidelines and practice parameters recommend the initial use of monotherapy whenever possible. Because large sample sizes are needed to determine whether one AED is superior to another in achieving seizure control, there have been very few 'head-to-head' randomised controlled trials (RCTs). Therefore, most comparative trials demonstrate only equal efficacy. Trials have demonstrated in the pediatric/adolescent age group that clobazam, phenytoin and carbamazepine are equally effective (17) and the same when topiramate, carbamazepine and valproate monotherapy were compared with each other (18). A recent and direct large 'head-to-head' trial has suggested that sodium valproate is more effective than lamotrigine or topiramate in treating generalized and unclassifiable seizures (9). The same study suggested that carbamazepine and lamotrigine were almost equally effective in treating partial seizures, although lamotrigine was slightly better tolerated, with fewer side effects; both of these drugs were more effective than oxcarbazepine, topiramate and gabapentin (19).

Initial monotherapy leads to success in approximately 60% of cases, although this will vary depending on the specific epilepsy syndrome. However, if seizures persist or there are significant adverse side effects, the next step will be to replace or substitute the first drug with a second first- or second-line drug. Once the second drug has been increased to an adequate or maximum-tolerated dose, and seizure control is achieved, then it would be appropriate to try and gradually withdraw the first drug.

If the second drug is unhelpful, either the first or second drug should be reduced and discontinued; which drug is discontinued will depend on their relative efficacies, side effects and tolerability, before starting another drug.

Prior to using combination therapy the clinician should reconsider the original diagnosis of epilepsy, but also the nature of any new paroxysmal episodes, to ensure that the diagnosis is accurate. There should also be an assessment of the young person's compliance or adherence with the medication; this is a relatively common cause of apparent poor seizure control. A reassessment of the choice of AED is also useful to ensure that appropriate medication options have been tried; this may also improve adherence with the prescribed medication if the new drug is better tolerated. Although routine anticonvulsant level monitoring is not recommended, it may be helpful to assess the young person's adherence at this point. Combination therapy is also indicated if a specific epilepsy syndrome has been identified which responds better to a combination regime, or if seizures are frequent and intrusive despite a trial of two or, at most, three appropriate drugs used as monotherapy.

Many of the antiepileptic drugs prescribed for children in both the UK and North America do not have a licence for use in adolescence or may have a licence but not for the intended epilepsy indication (called 'off label' use). These regulatory issues often require discussion with families and the child's family doctor or general practitioner. The Royal College of Pediatrics and Child health (RCPCH) recommend that informed use of unlicenced medication is often required (and justified) in pediatric practice. The RCPCH has produced supporting documentation on this issue for clinicians to share with families (see: www.medicinesforchildren.org).

There is evidence of potential differences in bioavailability between generic and proprietary (branded) forms of the same anticonvulsant drug. It is recommended that when a young person is started on a particular brand (ideally) or generic preparation, they should remain on that preparation. Although there may be cost differences, these are outweighed by potential changes in efficacy or tolerability, or both, when changing to a different product.

At the time of initial diagnosis, discussion with the patient and family about the expected duration of treatment is important. Once seizure-free, the management plan will include a discussion about discontinuation of an AED before the adolescent or family does it spontaneously and abruptly, with potentially serious consequences. A large meta-analysis found that the overall chances of remaining seizure-free after one to five years of seizure freedom appear to be 60–70% (20). There are several pediatric studies which address the issue of duration of treatment. In a Canadian series of 97 children and adolescents, 66% successfully discontinued their AED after 12 months of seizure freedom (21). A Dutch study randomized 161 children whose epilepsy was controlled within two months of treatment to four additional months of treatment (total treatment time six months) *versus* ten additional months of treatment (total treatment time 12 months) (22). The success rate in the six-month group was 45% compared with 51% in the 12-month group. In a Swedish study, children were randomized at the time of diagnosis to receive one year or three years of treatment; the success rate in the one-year treatment group was 53% compared with 71% in the three-year group (23). We conclude that two and no more than three years of seizure freedom is associated with a lower relapse rate than six or 12 months of seizure freedom. An additional meta-analysis reviewed seven trials comprising 924 children and came to the same conclusion, namely that the risk of seizure-recurrence is greater with less than two years of seizure freedom (20). In our view, the literature suggests that if seizures are easily controlled with monotherapy, treatment beyond two years of seizure freedom is usually unnecessary. The UK's NICE guidelines consider a two-year seizure-free period as the optimal for drug withdrawal. At this point, 60–70% will remain seizure-free off medication.

There is no firm evidence to define the time period over which a drug should be withdrawn (24). The relapse rates are similar for withdrawal over six weeks and withdrawal over nine months, although these data are quite old (25). Most clinicians in the UK would taper an AED over two to three months but some medications such as benzodiazepines or phenobarbital may require a much longer, more gradual taper. In North America the taper is often completed after several weeks.

The age at which a young person wishes to attempt drug withdrawal is also crucial. At a time in their life when they are looking to achieve qualifications, consider higher education or employment, obtaining a driving licence or move out of the family home, young people are concerned about the implications that further seizures may have on their plans. Consequently, many would prefer to remain on an AED to try to realise their ambitions. Conversely, other young people profoundly dislike having to take medication (for many reasons) and will opt for discontinuation at the first opportunity. The ultimate decision is highly individual and the clinician's role is to provide the young person with all the available facts and information to help them make their decision and also to support them through any subsequent period of withdrawal, particularly enabling rapid medical access should they relapse. Over 50% of relapses occur within the first six months, and 80–90% by two years, following discontinuation of medication.

For the 30–40% who relapse, it is very unusual for them not to regain complete seizure control again following reinstatement of their previous treatment and long-term remission is possible after a further treatment period (of at least two or more years). However, the risk of a subsequent relapse is thought to be higher than at the time of the first attempted AED withdrawal. Although there are no randomized trials, population-based cohorts have demonstrated that an additional 40% will again remain seizure-free. The relapse rate is higher after a two-year seizure-free period for those with an identified cause for their epilepsy, or children aged over 12 years at the onset of their epilepsy. An abnormal EEG at the time of discontinuation is also associated with a slightly higher relapse rate. In practice an EEG is rarely done as the findings would often not change the planned clinical action, from the perspective of both the patient and doctor. Some epilepsy syndromes including JME have much higher rates of seizure relapse on drug withdrawal and counseling on drug discontinuation must take this into account.

Adherence issues

Taking a daily medication is difficult for everyone, but especially for those in the early or middle part of adolescence – the time of life when they are seeking to become independent and 'take control.' The early years are concerned with the 'here and now' along with peer acceptance and only gradually evolve into the ability of abstract thinking of cause and effect and eventual independence (26). To the adolescent there is much more to life than epilepsy and tablets. Because of the random occurrence of seizures, when non-adherence happens and medication is forgotten or deliberately missed, it does not mean that the epilepsy has 'gone'. The most common reason for an increase in seizure frequency in this age group is poor adherence. One of the major reasons for non-adherence with medication generally results from the parents' or the clinician's opinion or 'recommendation' that an AED is mandatory; the teenager is often given no say in the matter, or perceives that their voice and opinion are not heard. Life for teenagers is complicated, busy and often unplanned and everyone wants to be 'normal' – and importantly, perceived as being 'normal.' Consequently it should be expected that at some time, young people will omit their medication. In addition, most adolescents would admit that the omission of one or more doses of their AED will serve as a 'test' to disprove the continued need for an AED and establish their 'normal' status. Clinicians need to recognize that poor adherence will be relatively common at this time of life; it is also important that they respond appropriately and do not adopt an accusatory or off-hand manner.

Other than the obvious need for education about the seizure disorder and the role of an AED in suppressing seizures there must also be a management plan in place for any recurrence. This might include monitoring the duration of a seizure, avoiding injury, relaxing or sleeping after the seizure, calling parents, the use of rescue medication and visiting/phoning their clinician or epilepsy nurse specialist. The following may also be helpful for the young person:

- finding a regular time for medication, yet one which is flexible enough to fit into a busy teenager's schedule. Whatever the teenager always does first thing in the morning and last thing in the evening should be the times that they take their medication
- using a 7-day pill box as a visual reminder (and parents can check themselves rather than asking all the time, which really annoys the teenager)
- carrying a few tablets in a wallet or backpack when away from home
- taking the medication before going out for a late night or sleepover
- asking the teenager if they have developed any obvious and upsetting side effects from their AED, and if so, consider changing the formulation or even the drug.

Restrictions

Restrictions are only those necessary to minimize stigma and injury, and to encourage the adolescent's development. Too many restrictions can potentially limit independence and exacerbate behavioral or psychosocial dysfunction. These problems may then persist into adulthood *(see the ILAE Commission Report in Epilepsia 1997; 38: 1054–56)*.

Triggers

Most people with epilepsy will not be able to identify a specific trigger for their seizures. However, there are some well-recognized triggers and these are more likely to occur during adolescence, although they may occur at other ages. These include poor adherence to an AED regime, menstruation, sleep deprivation, photic stimulation and stress. Improvement in seizure control by non-pharmacological treatments or adjustment in lifestyle in young people is worth attempting although there is no published evidence to support these lifestyle measures. Specific issues include the following:

Avoidance of provocative stimuli: Seizures in some epilepsy syndromes that predominate in early adolescence (often around the time of puberty) are clearly provoked by specific stimuli. Juvenile myoclonic epilepsy is associated with EEG photosensitivity in at least 30% and perhaps as much as 60% of cases, but only rarely does an environmental flashing light actually precipitate a seizure. The following may reduce the likelihood of a photically induced seizure:

- advice to cover one eye completely in the presence of flashing lights (this is because it requires binocular input for a photo-myoclonic or photo-convulsive response)
- to sit at least three feet from the television screen, using a remote control, and increase the background lighting in the room
- computers also should be used in a well-lit room, with good distance (at least 18 inches) from the screen
- to use dark, polarized sunglasses in sunlight
- to try and avoid situations that have high-frequency flickering or stroboscopic lights. Flicker frequency of most stroboscopic lights at dances tends to be < 10 Hz, which is below the frequencies that usually induce seizures (12–30 Hz).

Other, non-photically induced reflex epilepsies – which are very rare – usually have specific triggers that are difficult to avoid, including reading, communication, eating, music, bathing or mental calculations.

Sleep-deprivation: Many people with epilepsy note that moderate or severe lack of sleep precipitates their seizures. Almost every adolescent enjoys staying up late for many reasons – studying, talking on the phone, watching television or just 'chilling-out.' These are such normal activities that they are difficult to avoid. The use of excessive alcohol may readily exacerbate sleep-deprivation. If it is clear that a certain amount of sleep is critical for seizure control, then a 'guideline' based on fact may be useful. A regular sleep pattern and trying to avoid deviating from this pattern by more than two hours may reduce the risk of a seizure. A sleep calendar may be of help. A late night should be anticipated with the opportunity to 'sleep in' the next morning or perhaps take an 'afternoon nap' before the late night. Frequently, teenagers are employed outside school hours. Working more than 15 hours per week, especially with evening or night shifts, may not be compatible with adequate sleep to prevent seizures and should be avoided.

Stress: The ability for excessive stress to provoke a seizure is well known anecdotally to both physicians and families. However, there are no studies in the medical literature which actually prove this point. All information is derived from self-perception of seizure precipitants from questionnaire studies on adults. Stress is the most commonly reported seizure-precipitating feature, noted in 30–83%, depending on the population studied. It is possible that stress may exert an indirect effect by impairing sleep, or increasing alcohol intake, or both and it may be these factors which lead to breakthrough seizures. It is unclear if stress reduction improves seizure control; however, the goal is intuitively worthwhile, whatever its mechanism of action. In addition, using biofeedback and other behavior modification techniques can improve health-related quality of life both in teen-agers and adults.

Alcohol, recreational drugs and alternative therapies: In most countries, alcohol use is not legal in the early and mid-teenage years, although its use is highly prevalent. It is our impression that many clinicians fail to enquire about alcohol use in their teenage patients. In adults, there is good evidence that social drinking such as one or two glasses of wine or bottles of beer in an evening has no effect on seizure control. Adolescent alcohol-use is often excessive and its effect on epilepsy control is unclear. However, excessive use may impair the efficacy of antiepileptic medication and impair sleep. It is important that adolescents are given factual information and explanations as to why excessive alcohol may lower the threshold for further seizures so that they can make their own decisions. Methods can also be suggested to explain to their friends why they do not want to drink excessively, including diluting their drinks or drinking any alcohol slowly over an evening, or volunteering to be the 'designated driver' for friends.

Animal and human research on the effects of marijuana on seizure activity has shown inconclusive findings in patients with epilepsy. There are currently insufficient data to determine whether occasional or chronic marijuana use influences seizure frequency at any age. Some evidence suggests that marijuana and its active cannabinoids have antiepileptic effects, but these may be specific to partial or tonic-clonic seizures.

Both alcohol and marijuana use can transiently impair short-term memory which may lead to poor adherence with AEDs. Their use is often associated with sleep-deprivation, which compounds the effect. Case series have indicated that both alcohol and marijuana may potentially trigger seizures in susceptible patients during acute withdrawal of the drug. Other 'recreational' drugs including cocaine and ecstasy do lower seizure-threshold.

Sexuality and contraceptive usage: It is entirely appropriate, if not wise, for clinicians to discuss and educate children about sexuality both before and during puberty. Sexual activity is common in young teenagers and pregnancies do occur. Specific issues do need to be discussed with these young people and because many of these issues are sensitive and are best discussed outside the hospital clinic this emphasizes the invaluable role of the nurse specialist in epilepsy. These topics include (27, 28):

- the influence of the menstrual cycle on seizure frequency and severity (see below)
- the rarity of infertility in women with epilepsy
- an explanation for why consistent adherence to AEDs is necessary
- the fact that women with epilepsy can become pregnant with or without AEDs
- the importance of planning a pregnancy and the referral of young people to a specific pre-conception clinic with expert advice from specialists in both epilepsy and obstetrics
- the role of genetics associated with some epilepsy syndromes – and providing some idea of the risk of epilepsy occurring in their children
- the recognized teratogenicity of AEDs and the need to optimize the AED regime for a planned pregnancy
- the need for effective and consistent contraception to avoid an unplanned pregnancy
- effective contraception choices and possible contraceptive failure with specific antiepileptic drugs (e.g., carbamazepine, topiramate, high-dose lamotrigine, phenytoin) and the need to consider a barrier method for added protection
- the need for a calcium supplement and vitamin D for bone health
- the possible value of folate supplementation (5 mg per day) to reduce the risk of neural tube defects.

During the three years after onset of menstruation, menses are normally irregular and infrequent. This is a major reason why catamenial epilepsy (increase in the seizure frequency or pattern, or both, associated with the menstrual cycle) is only occasionally noted at puberty-onset and during the early and middle years of adolescence. Catamenial epilepsy is thought to be related to the variation in neuroactive properties of estradiol and progesterone during the menstrual cycle, but the underlying mechanism and treatment remains unclear. The exact frequency of catamenial epilepsy is unclear with the most systematic studies suggesting that the menstrual cycle increases seizure frequency at least two-fold in approximately one-third (35%) of women with epilepsy.

Specific issues that should be discussed with males include:

- the role of genetics associated with some epilepsy syndromes – and providing some idea of the risk of epilepsy occurring in their children
- the need for effective and consistent contraception to avoid an unplanned pregnancy
- the issues of decreased libido, erectile dysfunction and impotence or infertility are complex and infrequent. Counseling should be individualized for boys and young men. Up to 40% of males with epilepsy have low levels of free testosterone, which stimulates the development of male sex organs, sexual traits and sperm. Low testosterone may result in delayed sexual development with decreased testicular volume, penile length, and delayed pubic hair staging. The mechanism for low testosterone is perhaps because of increased metabolism from enzyme-inducing AEDs (phenobarbital, carbamazepine, oxcarbazepine, phenytoin, valproate, and topiramate). Combination therapy (polytherapy) appears to be associated with a greater risk of delayed puberty and low testosterone levels. Epilepsy itself, particularly temporal lobe epilepsy, may also have an adverse effect on male reproductive function with reduced libido and fertility. This implies a possible effect of seizures on the hypothalamic–pituitary–testicular axis, although data are very limited. Lastly, but no less importantly, higher levels of anxiety, depression and psychological distress are correlated with sexual dysfunction. It is therefore very unlikely that abnormal hormone levels *per se* are the primary cause of sexual dysfunction in males with epilepsy.

Treatment of the partial and progressive myoclonic epilepsies

Focal (partial) epilepsy

Pediatricians and pediatric neurologists have for many years preferred carbamazepine to sodium valproate as the first-line treatment for focal-onset seizures. However, randomized controlled studies have shown little difference in efficacy or tolerability (largely interpreted as the incidence of side effects) in the two treatments. There does appear to be a small advantage for carbamazepine when comparing 12-month remission rates, a finding supported by a recent meta-analysis (29). A comparative randomized and blinded trial undertaken in Canadian children and adolescents found equal efficacy between carbamazepine, clobazam and phenytoin after 12 months treatment (17).

Following the introduction in the 1990s of several new AEDs licensed for previously drug resistant focal epilepsies, the question was obviously raised as to whether carbamazepine remained the first-choice AED. Data on these new AEDs were largely derived from studies on previously drug resistant adult patients in relatively small numbers of patients and with short follow-up periods; in addition, many of the licensing studies compared the new AED with placebo, which clearly does not reflect 'real life.'

The largest 'head-to-head' comparative study, the SANAD study, published in 2007, attempted to address the question of which AED was the best initial treatment (19). A total of 1721 patients with newly diagnosed epilepsy (including 376 under the age of 16 [20%]), for whom the treating clinician would have normally started carbamazepine, were randomized to treatment with carbamazepine, gabapentin, lamotrigine, oxcarbazepine or topiramate. Using efficacy and tolerability outcome measures, the study showed a small advantage for lamotrigine over carbamazepine; the slight advantage was primarily because of the better tolerability of lamotrigine (fewer patients withdraw from this drug), than carbamazepine. Oxcarbazepine was 'third' and all three drugs demonstrated a significant benefit over both gabapentin and topiramate.

The study was, predictably, subject to some criticism; a few pediatric neurologists felt that the results could not be extrapolated to children because of the relatively low proportion of adolescents in the sample and a small number of specific epilepsy syndromes. This was in contrast to the majority who felt that the results were valid and reflected clinical practice, largely because it is the seizure type (and not necessarily the specific epilepsy syndrome) that is important, and most AEDs are chosen on the basis of the seizure type. In the individual patient there may be specific reasons for preferring one AED to the other and this is often based on any potential adverse effects or interactions with other medications (i.e., the effect of the oral contraceptive pill on both lamotrigine and carbamazpine).

Most new antiepileptic drugs are developed for use in people (typically adults) with focal epilepsy with or without secondary generalization; therefore most of these drugs gain a licence for this indication, initially as adjunctive treatment, and subsequently often as monotherapy. With time and increasing experience with these drugs, their licence may be expanded for other seizure types, including those that occur in generalized epilepsies. Consequently, other drugs may be used if either lamotrigine or carbamazepine is ineffective or poorly tolerated. These usually include clobazam, levetiracetam, oxcarbazepine or topiramate and if these are ineffective or not tolerated, gabapentin (poor efficacy), lacosamide, sodium valproate, tiagabine (again, limited efficacy), vigabatrin and zonisamide. The specific choice will be determined by both the drug's safety profile and the personal experience and preference of the clinician.

Acetazolamide is occasionally tried as adjunctive therapy, although the evidence for its use is very limited. Acetazolamide may be effective when used with carbamazepine in the treatment of focal seizures and rarely with sodium valproate in resistant idiopathic generalized (absence or myoclonic) seizures.

There is evidence that the ketogenic diet may be effective in up to 30% of children with focal epilepsies who are resistant to at least two AEDs. However, most variants of the ketogenic diet (even the modified Atkins variant) are rarely acceptable in adolescence and there is little evidence for its benefit in this age group.

Progressive myoclonic epilepsies

Sodium valproate, levetiracetam and the benzodiazepines are the AEDs that are most commonly used in treating these difficult epilepsies and those that show the greatest efficacy. Piracetam has a very limited spectrum of action and its use is largely restricted to adjunctive treatment with sodium valproate or levetiracetam in the suppression of the myoclonic seizures but also the non-epileptic myoclonus that frequently occurs in many of these disorders. It is important to avoid phenytoin because this drug may exacerbate not only the myoclonic seizures but may accelerate the cognitive decline and dementia in most of the PMEs.

There are clearly many available AED options when treating adolescents with epilepsy and to try all options may take quite a few years. Important data about adults with epilepsy that hadn't responded to drug treatment was published by Kwan and Brodie in 2000 (30). This study suggested that if the first drug fails only about 10% will achieve seizure freedom with a second medication. A single population-based study in children indicated a better outcome (40%) but in either case, failure of a first drug is discouraging. Trial of a second or third drug as monotherapy is still indicated. The value of combination therapy (polytherapy) has not been systematically assessed but is often attempted when several trials of monotherapy have been ineffective. Considerable anecdotal experience suggests that the two AEDs used in combination in people whose seizures were uncontrolled on monotherapy, may result in approximately 10–15% becoming seizure-free.

Non-drug options should be considered once the first two or three antiepileptic drugs have failed to control the epilepsy. These include the ketogenic diet, surgery or vagal nerve stimulation (VNS). When the prognosis of the young person's epilepsy is discussed with the family, and if this is likely to be poor, it is important to try and maintain hope for the young person's future and confidence in the role of medical treatment. This may take several consultations not only in hospital but also in the home, which is a specific responsibility (and strength) of the epilepsy nurse specialist. This is often the point when the family becomes more acutely aware of the potential of the future for the young person. A second opinion on the diagnostic aspects but also management of the teenager's epilepsy should be sought at this stage, as recommended by NICE and SIGN.

Epilepsy surgery

The assessment for epilepsy surgery must be undertaken in a specialized centre by a team that is experienced in assessing children for surgery. In addition to high-resolution MRI, additional, functional neuro-imaging may be needed including functional MRI and ictal or inter-ictal nuclear medicine scans (SPECT) or positron emission tomography (PET). Functional MRI is likely to become more developed and therefore of more practical use over the next few years and will probably replace the need for SPECT and other invasive methods used to assess language and memory function. Video–EEG to include ictal recordings of habitual seizures is essential; this sometimes necessitates drug reduction or even temporary discontinuation. The video allows comparison of the semiology with the historical description as well as the identification of the site of electrical seizure onset. Occasionally invasive video–EEG telemetry will be required for both precise localization of seizure onset but also to undertake stimulation of the cortex adjacent to the lesion;

this is not only to define the extent of any resection but also to avoid the resection of importantly eloquent cortex, which might result in an irreversible motor or speech and language deficit.

Detailed neuro-psychological and neuropsychiatric assessments are usually needed to evaluate the level of functioning and lateralization of specific skills, specifically language and memory. This allows some prediction of what functions may be affected by resective surgery and whether further investigative assessments are needed, such as functional MRI (fMRI) or Wada-testing. The psychiatric assessment establishes a baseline as mood and emotion disorders may occur post-surgery and provides a semi-independent view of whether the family has under-stood the important issues around epilepsy surgery and also their expectations.

One of the key issues in epilepsy surgery is to consider its viability early and whether the teenager's focal epilepsy may be treatable (including curable) with resective surgery. Focal seizures arising for the first time in a child aged > 14 years, particularly from sleep, should raise the possibility that there may be an underlying structural cause, including a tumor. It is recommended that epilepsy surgery be considered if there is any focal abnormality on MRI or even in those with multiple focal abnormalities. If focal seizures remain uncontrolled after adequate doses of two appropriate antiepileptic drugs, or seizures continue two years after diagnosis (even if the MRI has been reported as normal), epilepsy surgery should be con-sidered and the patient referred to a specialist pediatric epilepsy surgery centre (14). The decision as to whether surgery is appropriate can only be made by a specialist team. The current evidence suggests that many people who are candidates for epilepsy surgery are not referred – perhaps as many as 75% in the UK and North America. It is of interest that detailed assessments are performed in three times as many patients as are operations performed. There are also specific epilepsy syn-dromes which, although relatively rare, have a considerably better long-term out-come with surgical rather than medical treatment, but only when referred early in their natural history. Specific examples include Rasmussen's syndrome and Sturge–Weber syndrome. Reluctance to refer children and adolescents for consideration of epilepsy surgery is based on misconceptions about the dangers of the procedures. Most surgical procedures in specialist centres are associated with a very low mor-bidity and a success rate of at least > 50%. It is important to understand that the following situations are not contraindications to performing a surgical evaluation or indeed a surgical procedure:

- the apparent absence of a lesion on conventional MRI
- a seizure onset in what appears to be the dominant hemisphere
- the presence of learning or behavior difficulties, or both.

The most common site for epilepsy surgery is the temporal lobe. Medial temporal lobe surgery, whether a selective anterior temporal resection or more selective amygdalo-hippocampectomy, will result in long-term seizure freedom in around 60–80% of young people. Other surgical procedures including extra-temporal (usually frontal) focal resections, lobar resections and hemi-spherectomy (removal of one cerebral hemisphere) or hemispherotomy (disconnection of the hemisphere but the cerebrum is left *in situ*), are associated with lower success rates but still may render more than 50% of patients long-term seizure-free. A detailed discussion of epilepsy surgery is beyond the scope of this text, but the key point is that it must never be regarded as a treatment option of 'last resort.' Young people with a focal epilepsy should be referred at an early stage for specialist assessment within an established epilepsy surgical program.

Finally, vagal nerve stimulation can be considered in those young people with drug resistant epilepsy in whom a surgical resection is either not possible or unacceptable. It remains unclear as to which particular seizure types and epilepsy syndromes respond best to VNS. Considerable anecdotal but no significant randomized controlled data seem to suggest that this therapy might be effective for patients with both partial and generalized seizures. Unlike the response to antiepileptic drugs, the benefit of VNS may not be seen for many months following its insertion. The vast majority of patients in whom VNS proves effective still seem to require at least one AED for long-term seizure control. Finally, complications of VNS-insertion are infrequent and include hoarseness (usually transient), infection, and fracture of the electrode, usually in the neck. The battery life in the latest generation of stimulators is usually seven years, although this can vary depending upon the settings and use of the magnet, which can be swiped across the stimulator to try and shorten or even abort a seizure.

Cognitive and social outcomes in later years for IGEs and partial epilepsies

Predictors of the cognitive and social outcomes of adolescents with epilepsy are related to the epilepsy itself, its treatment, the underlying lesion, co-morbidity and additional health issues, and personal or perceived reactions to epilepsy (stigma). The level of cognition and health related co-morbidities (e.g., ADHD, asthma, migraine, depression, anxiety and physical disability) are important. Most studies have shown that more than 50% of adolescents have at least one co-morbidity, any one of which may increase the burden of epilepsy, which in itself is considerable and may result from many factors:

- seizure control
- AED side effects, lifestyle restrictions
- economic burden
- peer or societal stigma.

Social and cognitive outcome of juvenile myoclonic epilepsy

It has long been considered that people with JME tend to have a recognized clinical phenotype including being impulsive, immature and irresponsible, which may directly contribute to poor seizure control (12). They were said to have, 'an engaging, but emotionally unstable, fairly immature personality, wavering between camaraderie and mistrust, which may lead to difficulties in social adaption.'. These features had not been re-evaluated until relatively recently. In a population-based study of children in Nova Scotia with new-onset JME and with a 20-year follow-up, approximately 70% reported good satisfaction with their health, work, friendships and social life. However, despite the fact that 87% had graduated from high school, 31% were unemployed at the end of follow-up. Forty percent received antidepressants and many perceived themselves as anxious and socially isolated. Seventy percent were living with a partner. Although 60% had experienced at least one pregnancy, 80% of these pregnancies had been unplanned and outside a stable relationship. At least one major unfavorable social outcome was noted in 76% of the cohort (12).

Recent systematic studies find that patients with JME have neuro-psychological deficits which suggest frontal lobe dysfunction. In addition, neuro-diagnostic imaging studies have indicated problems arising from the frontal area. Although comparison of JME patients with controls using the Minnesota Multiphasic Personality Inventory (MMPI) fails to show a specific profile for JME, other studies have found a range of psychiatric disorders to be associated with JME.

Social and cognitive outcome of the focal epilepsies

The social outcome of children with focal (partial) epilepsy has been studied primarily in case series of specific focal epilepsy syndromes and usually from specialized tertiary epilepsy clinic populations. There is little literature on the long-term psychosocial or cognitive health of adolescents with newly diagnosed focal epilepsy or for those with focal epilepsy that has persisted from childhood into adolescence.

Similarly, the frequency of behavioral problems is not based on information available from population-based studies but on relatively small cohorts in children with a wide range of ages and abilities, including adolescents. Methodology to evaluate adolescent behavior problems is not well developed, including neuro-psychological testing batteries. Attention-related problems and impulsivity are often noted, as well as internalizing behaviors in non-lesional epilepsies (i.e., cryptogenic). Other abnormal behaviors in focal epilepsy are thought to be related to the location of the lesion. For example, adolescents with frontal lobe epilepsy may have impaired executive function, impulsivity and poor social judgment. Individuals with temporal lobe epilepsy may have memory problems and affective disorders, while those with parietal epilepsy may have visual processing problems leading to difficulty utilizing visual cues which occur during social interactions.

It is accepted that more than 50% of adolescents with persistent childhood-onset focal epilepsy have borderline cognitive abilities or 'mental retardation,' either of which may lead to a poor social outcome. For those with focal epilepsy diagnosed in the teenage years, there is no population-based information on the frequency of cognitive dysfunction, but it is our impression that cognition is affected to some degree in the majority.

Finally, epilepsy, whether focal or generalized, is often described as a 'hidden handicap' that can only be understood by others if they are told about it. Yet, one US study found that more than 50% of teenagers would not date someone with epilepsy, and often regarded epilepsy as a mental illness. This is not conducive to good psychosocial health in young people with epilepsy.

Suggestions for management of young people with epilepsy and cognitive or behavioral problems

Adolescents with epilepsy and cognitive difficulties frequently experience special difficulties. Most importantly, the presence or the degree of any learning difficulties or behavior problems may not have been recognized. In addition, even if such difficulties are identified, appropriate management may be poor or even absent. For example, the clinician may not have treated seizures of minor severity or may not have appreciated that the AED dose may have been too high. The family may be dysfunctional and/or chaotic and not have been able to respond to their child's needs. The school or community child health service may not have arranged a careful neuro-psychological assessment in an adolescent with a focal epilepsy (which may be associated with a specific, rather than general learning difficulty – as in a frontal or temporal lobe epilepsy). Society and the teenager's peers may stigmatize the young person with epilepsy as being unreliable or liable to mood swings or even violent outbursts. Consequently, it should not be surprising that these problems, within the context of the increasing demands of adolescent development, may result in either introversion (and social isolation or withdrawal) or extroversion (and delinquent or aggressive behavior). Both may subsequently adversely affect the young person's adherence with medication and medical contact, with a spiraling of any psychopathology.

There remains though a vigorous debate among epilepsy neurologists as to whether better control of inter-ictal EEG abnormalities could improve cognitive outcome. Aldenkamp created a predictive model encompassing the effects of epilepsy on cognition and educational achievement (31). The underlying brain pathology is assumed to be responsible for both the development of seizures and cognitive impairment. In addition, the frequency of EEG epileptiform discharges (specifically spike and wave activity) and seizures together with possible antiepileptic treatment effects may impair concentration or memory (or both) and contribute to any cognitive difficulties. It is a relatively common phenomenon in epilepsy clinics to see children who appeared to have coped well in mainstream education at a primary level but who then start to demonstrate increasing difficulties in secondary education. Although cognitive progress is usually made, it may be a slower rate than most of their classmates, and the gap between the adolescent and their peers widens. Educational under-achievement frequently ensues with adverse effects on their further education, career potential and social development.

It is therefore crucial that young people with epilepsy have access to services where the outcomes of these interactions are well understood. The education and training of teachers and psychologists and appropriate support services including child and adolescent mental health services (CAMHS) are essential to recognize, diagnose and hopefully minimize or even prevent the development of behavioural problems and poor social outcomes in later adulthood. This requires adequately trained – and numbers – of professionals, organized into networks of care to support the young person with epilepsy.

Transition of teenagers to adult epilepsy services

There are two unique groups of adolescents that must be considered separately – those that have relatively normal intelligence and those with severe difficulties.

Young people with relatively normal intelligence

It is not easy for young people to navigate adolescence successfully with chronic epilepsy. Restrictions are frequently in place: regular sleep hours, adherence to medication, no alcohol, and some limitation of activities (particularly driving), and uncertainty about contraceptive efficacy for girls.

During childhood and early adolescence, epilepsy care is family-focused. Adult epilepsy care tends to be focused on the individual. As a child, it is the parents who ensure that medication is not forgotten and who suggest a regular bedtime and carefully supervised lifestyle. The clinician usually concurs with this approach. As an adult, the person takes control and makes his or her own choices. The consequences of poor compliance or poor lifestyle choices may not be understood. The clinician who treats adults (and particularly if not a neurologist) may not seem to care once the initial diagnosis has been disclosed and management discussed and will then leave the patient on their own – to make good or bad decisions.

The 'transfer' of young people from pediatric to adult epilepsy care is potentially sudden and may be brutal. The adolescent, now overnight perceived to be an adult, does not understand their epilepsy. Previous discussion and decision-making will have been directed towards the family and will have been many years earlier. The adult epileptologist is likely only to be provided with a case summary and is unlikely to fully appreciate how much of a burden epilepsy is to an adolescent, even if the seizures are well controlled. In addition the clinic environment and clinic staff will be very different between a pediatric department or children's hospital and an adult clinic in a large hospital. This may be quite intimidating for the 17- or 18-year-old. In contrast, the 'transition' from pediatric to adult care is conceptually more attractive and, by definition, must be a dynamic process.

'Transition' means that the young person and their family and adult epileptologist will all learn the critical steps to enable the teenager with epilepsy to be treated in the adult world. Transition is a process that takes time and needs to begin in the pediatric clinic, probably from the age of 13 or 14 years, possibly earlier. The adolescent learns what they need to know to not only understand and explain their disorder, but also take control – a process often termed 'self-empowerment.' They learn the names of the drugs, the doses, the side effects and what needs to be done to fill a prescription. They understand that they have epilepsy but are not 'epileptic.' They learn that for most young people with epilepsy it is far more about what they can do, rather than what they can't do, which is so important for their confidence and self-esteem. 'Transitional' epilepsy care can be undertaken in many ways and formats; there is no evidence to support which is likely to be the most effective – for the young person and their family. Intuitively, we believe that the needs of these young people are best addressed by a transition clinic which is staffed by both adult and pediatric epilepsy specialists, with nurse specialist support. Regular reviews in this transition clinic should take place until transfer to adult care is considered appropriate. The family will be reassured that their child's pediatrician or pediatric neurologist will remain involved as part of this transitional or 'hand-over' clinic until communication with the adult team is complete and the young person is ready and confident to move on to the adult service. The adult team needs to understand at what stage the particular adolescent is in the process of becoming an adult and adopt an approach that is appropriate for that individual. A key component of the art of the transitional process is facilitating the family, and specifically the teenager's parents, to 'separate' from their child and allow them to take responsibility and control of their epilepsy; this is often very difficult for the family and very occasionally they will need support, as much support as the young person themselves (26, 32).

Young people with severe learning difficulties

It is important to appreciate that approximately 50% of epilepsy that begins in childhood and persists into adulthood is accompanied by significant learning difficulties, including mental handicap. The situation is therefore more complex when the young person has significant learning difficulties. The parents and guardians have an ongoing supervisory role and the young person is generally followed up by an epilepsy specialist; it is important that these specialists have the necessary understanding and skills to manage any co-morbidities.

Pediatric epilepsy specialists should have a relatively good understanding of how much independent judgment young people have and how likely they will be able to take decisions themselves. This is likely to be far more difficult for the adult neurologist. The individual-focused adult healthcare system may not be able to cope with young people and adults with epilepsy and severe learning difficulties because they will not be able to represent themselves completely. Unfortunately it is relatively common for clinicians to fail to take responsibility not only for the person's epilepsy but also their learning difficulties; consequently the family and the young person may feel unwanted and uncared for.

Parents will have invested many years of confidence and trust in the care of their child and, subsequently, their adolescent within the pediatric healthcare system and will need to be convinced that the adult system is equally caring and responsive. Unfortunately, experience has shown that this is the exception and certainly not the rule. Parents quickly recognize when things are not going well but they may not know how to address the problem. Access to, and seeking advice from, their child's epilepsy specialist may be very difficult and this can lead to distress and frustration. In certain situations the family may feel unable to cope and, coupled with a relative lack of support from adult healthcare services, may yield their responsibility to someone else, a guardian or foster family or a residential institution. Consequently, the transition is far more of a problem for the parents and the family than for the young person. The adult physician has few models and little experience in this area. Adult neurologists will often state that they have no problem with the young person (either in terms of their epilepsy or their personality), but they were unable to deal with their parents. If the child has severe learning difficulties (mental handicap), there is no escape from the parents. In our experience, parents of a mentally handicapped adolescent with chronic and poorly controlled epilepsy are often very reluctant to take adult neurology advice, and specifically the prescription of a new AED or discussion of a surgical procedure. They have come to accept a *status quo* that may be perceived as being 'difficult' or obstructive by the adult team.

The pediatrician and pediatric specialist also have to give up many years of medical care for the teenager and a long-standing relationship, and even bond with the family; breaking this bond may be equally difficult for the pediatrician. In this situation there is the temptation for the pediatrician or pediatric epilepsy specialist to continue caring for the young person until 18 or even 20 years of age. This is particularly relevant for those adolescents with severe learning difficulties. This is inappropriate for many reasons:

- the pediatrician is unlikely to have the required knowledge of adult-oriented social services and welfare benefits or the personal skills to manage young adults
- this practice will not facilitate the process of the young person becoming independent and taking responsibility, or their family 'separating' from their teenager
- if the young person requires hospitalization this will be to an adult unit or hospital with the junior doctors or residents and consultant having no knowledge of the person's epilepsy history or their treatment.

The social outcomes of young people with epilepsy, even with relatively normal intelligence, that persists into adulthood is unsatisfactory in 30–50%. For those young people with severe or profound learning difficulties, follow-up in the adult neurology services tends to be poor; specifically, newer AEDs are not prescribed and mental health issues may go unrecognised. In summary, the epilepsy community generally handles the 'transfer' or 'transition' of care to adult services poorly.

One possible solution must include the following:

- every pediatric epilepsy clinic – whether in a local hospital, tertiary hospital or specialist epilepsy unit – needs to identify one or more adult epilepsy specialists who are willing to participate in a structured transition clinic
- the transition clinic should be supervised by both a pediatric and an adult epilepsy specialist with support from an epilepsy nurse specialist
- the specialists should have knowledge about epilepsy and its investigation, all antiepileptic drugs, other treatment options, further education and employment issues, social integration and rehabilitation.

Clearly, such an approach does not guarantee success, but it does at least provide a model for genuine 'transitional' care; it would certainly represent an improvement compared to current practice.

The good news

The transition from childhood to young adulthood is an extraordinary period of testing limits and striving for independence through trial and error. Eventually moral and mature values develop along with an optimistic, rational but accepting approach to life with a chronic medical disorder.

This youthful stage is often challenging to healthcare providers and families. However, when ill-advised, unexpected or potentially dangerous adolescent activity does occur, it is often motivated by exploration and the search for self-identity, rather than because they want to cause trouble. At this age, most do not want to be different from their peers. Therefore, medication is 'forgotten', late hours or excessive alcohol intake or both are indulged in 'for a party,' or an over-the-counter medication is used which interferes with the metabolism of the prescribed AED.

It would seem wise for parents or carers to anticipate these behaviors and influence their child before puberty, so that the child grows to understand 'cause and effect' in their own behavior and is thereby able to make appropriate, independent decisions as a teenager. Clearly clinicians need to provide accurate factual information, advice and support and to show the family and the young person that they understand and are confident in the management of their epilepsy.

REFERENCES

1. Camfield C, Camfield PR, Gordon K, *et al.* Incidence of epilepsy in childhood and adolescence: a population based study in Nova Scotia form 1977–1985. *Epilepsia* 1996; **37**: 19–23.
2. Svalheim S, Taubøll E, Bjørnenak T, *et al.* Onset of epilepsy and menarche – is there any relationship? *Seizure* 2006; **15**: 571–5.
3. Diamantopoulos N, Crumrine PK. The effect of puberty on the course of epilepsy. *Arch Neurol* 1986; **43**: 873–6.
4. Stephenson JB. *Fits and Faints*. Philadelphia PA, MacKeith Press 1990.
5. Appleton RE. Psychogenic non-epileptic seizures. *Pediatric Epilepsy Current Awareness Service* 2006; **1**: 9–13.
6. Delagado-Escueta AV, Enrile-Bacsal F. Juvenile myoclonic epilepsy of Janz. *Neurology* 1984; **34**: 285–94.
7. Wirrell EC, Camfield CS, Camfield PR, Gordon K, Dooley J. Long-term prognosis of typical childhood absence epilepsy. *Neurology* 1996; **47**: 912–18.
8. Hirtz D, Berg A, Bettis D, *et al.* Practice parameter: The evaluation of a first nonfebrile seizure in children (an evidence-based review). Report of the Quality Standards Subcommittee of the American Academy of Neurology. *Neurology* 2000; **55**: 616–23.
9. Marson AG, Al-Kharusi, Alwaidh M, *et al.* SANAD Study Group. The SANAD study of effectiveness of valproate, lamotrigine or topiramate for treatment of generalized or unclassifiable epilepsy: an unblinded randomized controlled trial. *Lancet* 2007; **369**: 1016–26.
10. Nicolson A, Marson AG. When the first antiepileptic drug fails in a patient with juvenile myoclonic epilepsy. *Pract Neurol* 2010; **10**: 208–18.
11. Loddenkemper T, Benbadis SR, Serrasota JM, Berkovic SF. Idiopathic generalized epilepsy syndromes of childhood and adolescence. In: Wyllie E, ed. *The Treatment of Epilepsy Principles and Practice*. Philadelphia, PA, Lippincott Williams and Wilkins 2006; p. 296.

12. Camfield CS, Camfield PR. Juvenile myoclonic epilepsy 25 years after seizure onset: a population-based study. *Neurology* 2009; **73**: 1041–5.

13. Alving J, Beniczky S. Diagnostic usefulness and duration of the inpatient long-term video–EEG monitoring: findings in patients extensively investigated before the monitoring. *Seizure* 2010; **18**: 470–3.

14. National Institute for Health and Clinical Excellence (NICE). The epilepsies: the diagnosis and management of the epilepsies in adults and children in primary and secondary care. Clinical Guideline 20. *NICE* October 2004; www.nice.org.uk.

15. Scottish Intercollegiate Guidelines Network (SIGN). Diagnosis and management of epilepsies in children and young people Guideline 81. *SIGN* March 2005; www.sign.ac.uk.

16. Hirtz D, Berg A, Bettis D, *et al.* Practice parameter: treatment of the child with a first unprovoked seizure. Report of the Quality Standards Subcommittee of the American Academy of Neurology and Practice Committee of the Child Neurology Society. *Neurology* 2003; **60**: 166–75.

17. Canadian Study Group for Childhood Epilepsy. Clobazam has equivalent efficacy to carbamazepine and phenytoin as monotherapy for childhood epilepsy. *Epilepsia* 1998; **39**: 850–6.

18. Wheless JW and the EPMN-105 Study Group. Topiramate, carbamazepine, and valproate monotherapy: double-blind comparison in children with newly diagnosed epilepsy. *J Child Neurol* 2004; **19**: 135–41.

19. Marson AG, Al-Kharusi, Alwaidh M, *et al.* SANAD Study Group. The SANAD study of effectiveness of carbamazepine, gabapentin, lamotrigine, oxcarbazepine or topiramate for treatment of partial epilepsy: an unblinded randomised controlled trial. *Lancet* 2007; **369**: 1000–15.

20. Berg AT, Shinnar S. Relapse following discontinuation of antiepileptic drugs: meta-analysis. *Neurology* 1994; **44**: 601–8.

21. Dooley JM, Gordon K, Camfield PR, *et al.* Discontinuation of anticonvulsant therapy in children free of seizures for 1 year. *Neurology* 1996; **46**: 969–74.

22. Peters AC, Brouwer OF, Geerts AT, *et al.* Randomized prospective study of early discontinuation of AEDs in children with epilepsy. *Neurology* 1998; **50**: 724–30.

23. Braathen G, Anderson T, Gylie H, *et al.* A comparison between one and three years of treatment in uncomplicated childhood epilepsy: a prospective study. 1. Outcome in different seizure types. *Epilepsia* 1996; **37**: 822–32.

24. Ranganathian LN, Ramaratnam S. Rapid versus slow withdrawal of antiepileptic drugs. *Cochrane Database Syst Rev* 2006; **19**: CD005003.

25. Tennison M, Greenwood R, Lewis D, Thorn M. Discontinuing antiepileptic drugs in children with epilepsy: a comparison of a six-week and a nine-month taper. *N Engl J Med* 1994; **330**: 1407–10.

26. Appleton RE. Epilepsy in the teenager. *Paediatr Child Health* 2009; **19**: 232–5.

27. Harden CL, Pennell PB, Koppel BS, *et al.* Management issues for women with epilepsy – focus on pregnancy (an evidence-based review): II teratogenesis and perinatal outcomes. *Epilepsia* 2009; **50**: 1237–46.

28. Harden CL, Pennell PB, Koppel BS, *et al.* Management issues for women with epilepsy – focus on pregnancy (an evidence-based review): III vitamin K, folic acid, blood levels, and breast feeding. *Epilepsia* 2009; **50**: 1247–55.

29. Tudur-Smith C, Marson AG, Chadwick DW, Williamson PR. Multiple treatment comparisons in epilepsy monotherapy trials. *Trials* 2007; **8**: 34.

30. Kwan P, Brodie M. Early identification of refractory epilepsy. *N Engl J Med* 2000; **342**: 314–19.

31. Aldenkamp AP, Weber B, Overweg-Plandsoen WCG, Reijs R, van Mil S. Educational underachievement in children with epilepsy: a model to predict the effects of epilepsy on educational achievement. *J Child Neurol* 2005; **20**: 175–80.

32. Appleton RE, Chadwick D, Sweeney A. Managing the teenager with epilepsy: pediatric to adult care. *Seizure* 1997; **6**: 27–30.

5

Risks and hazards of epilepsy

Ingrid Tuxhorn and J. Helen Cross

Introduction

The Concise Oxford Dictionary defines a '*hazard*' as any situation that has a potential to cause damage or harm and a '*risk*' as the likelihood of a harm happening. Risks may in part be related to circumstances and the likelihood of the severity of the ensuing harm. All factors being equal, risks may be proportional to hazards; however risks are often multifactorial (e.g., genetic and acquired, even active in the same individual) and driven by probabilities that may contribute in a qualitative or quantitative way to harm.

The exact timing of seizures is rarely predictable and it is easy for families to perceive many potential and frightening hazards; however, very few studies have objectively defined the risks and hazards associated with childhood epilepsy. To guide us towards effective intervention and prevention, risk assessments in general terms need:

1) to identify the *source of potential hazards*, i.e., situations with potential to cause damage to the child with epilepsy
2) to determine the *likelihood or probability* that a particular hazard may happen to cause harm and
3) to determine the *severity and estimate the potential seriousness* of the harm that may be inflicted (the risk factors) (1).

This chapter will address:

a) the risks and hazards that are known to be closely related to seizure and epilepsy factors per se, including physical injury, mortality, seizure recurrences, likelihood of seizure remission, status epilepticus and problems related to the use of antiepileptic drugs (AEDs)

Childhood Epilepsy: Management from Diagnosis to Remission, ed. Richard Appleton and Peter Camfield. Published by Cambridge University Press. © Cambridge University Press 2011.

b) the risk factors related to the impact of seizures and epilepsy in the psychosocial arena, including risks for school and academic failure, cognitive dysfunction, behavior disorders and psychiatric morbidity, specifically depression.

Seizure-related risks and hazards

Physical injury and accidental death

Children and adolescents with epilepsy are at increased risk for accidents and injury. Based on a large European survey most accidents and associated injuries are minor and directly related to recurrent seizures or associated neurological disability or transient cognitive dysfunction (confusion) from the seizures and medication (2). Most accidents occur at home, in the street or at school or work. The types of injuries in decreasing frequency are contusions (bruises), wounds, abrasions, fractures, cerebral concussions, sprains/strains and burns. There is also a slightly higher risk for accidental death than in the general population. Causes for accidental death include burns, drowning, suffocation, aspiration of foreign bodies, falls and traffic-related accidents. In 1991, the Risks and Insurance Committee of the International Bureau of Epilepsy Commission on Epilepsy published baseline data that can help to guide patients, care-givers and physicians to reduce risk in different areas of daily life (3).

There are limited pediatric-specific data available on the risks of accidental injuries. Seizure type and severity have been consistently found to be risk factors for seizure-related injuries so that children with 'drop attacks' or a predominance of tonic-clonic seizures are at particular risk. Several reports suggest that wearing a helmet reduces the risk of head injury by one-third, although most studies suggest that these head injuries are minor. Wearing a helmet is obviously stigmatizing and should only be recommended for children who experience very frequent falls associated with 'drop' or tonic-clonic seizures. Children with absence seizures may also be at a higher risk for accidents. One population-based study suggested a risk of accidental injury of 9% per person per year, particularly bicycle accidents (4).

Death by drowning is four times more common in children with epilepsy than in the general population and most commonly occurs while the person is taking an unsupervised bath (5, 6). This has led to the recommendation that children with epilepsy should not take unsupervised baths, and a shower is a preferred alternative. There is some evidence suggesting that it is safe for children with epilepsy to swim with a friend in a lifeguard-supervised pool (5).

Although there are no data on which activities may constitute particular risks for children with epilepsy of different ages, a commonsense approach to risk assessment needs to be taken, remembering that there is a greater risk for accident-related injuries, that most injuries are mild and uncomplicated but that recurrence of seizures, associated disabilities and co-morbidities constitute a cumulative risk. Over-protection or a blanket restriction for all activities is inappropriate and should be avoided as they are likely to isolate and stigmatize the child with epilepsy.

Reducing risks and hazards with appropriate supervision should be the goal without imposing overly restrictive approaches that may prevent a child from leading as close to a normal life as possible.

Mortality risks and SUDEP

The risk of death (mortality rate) in patients with epilepsy is up to three times that in the general population. The causes may be the underlying cause of epilepsy, the seizures themselves (resulting in accidents [traffic-related, falling down stairs] or sudden unexpected death) or associated co-morbid conditions including physical and mental impairments that may be linked to epilepsy.

Sudden unexpected (or unexplained) death in epilepsy (SUDEP) is the leading cause of death in people with chronic and uncontrolled epilepsy, but it is rare in children. In fact, population-based studies of children with epilepsy have consistently demonstrated that those without significant neurological deficits have no increased risk of death compared to age-matched controls (7, 8). Children with severe neurological deficits have a very high mortality (25% within 20 years of epilepsy diagnosis) but the cause of death is almost never directly related to the seizures (7, 9) but to other (and often severe) medical co-morbidities.

The risk of SUDEP is highest in adults and children with refractory epilepsy and no particular epilepsy syndrome stands out except possibly Dravet syndrome (severe myoclonic epilepsy of infancy) (10, 11). Mortality prevention will need to focus on better control of seizures and improvements in the prevention or treatment of the underlying neurologic condition, a particularly difficult, if not impossible task in some patients. There is considerable debate about when the risk of death, including SUDEP, should be discussed with families (12, 13). Parents who have seen their child have a generalized tonic-clonic seizure nearly always worry that their child was actually dying, so that discussion of the risk of death is appropriate early in the context of overall risks of the epilepsy including treatment. It would appear that many physicians are reluctant to discuss SUDEP with families while the families expect to be offered, or are not overly alarmed by this information (13).

Risks for recurrence and remission of seizures

The most obvious risk for a child with epilepsy is for further seizures. Epilepsy begins with a first seizure; however, about one-half of children with a *first, unprovoked* afebrile seizure will not have any further seizures. One seminal study showed that those children who present with a first seizure without any known cause and have a normal EEG will have a particularly favorable prognosis, particularly when the seizure occurs while awake with a five-year recurrence risk of only about 21% (14). In a prospective study of 407 children with a first seizure, 42% experienced subsequent seizures and the cumulative risk of seizure recurrence was 29%, 37%, 42% and 44% at one, two, five and eight years respectively. The median time to recurrence was 5.7 months with 53% of recurrences occurring within six months,

69% within one year and 88% within two years. Only 3% of children experienced a recurrence after five years (15).

The risk factors for recurrence were:

- a remote symptomatic etiology (i.e., a defined previous brain abnormality)
- an abnormal EEG
- a seizure occurring during sleep
- a history of prior febrile seizures
- a Todd's paralysis (transient and unilateral weakness) when the cause was unknown and an abnormal EEG and occurrence from sleep remained risk factors for recurrence.

When two unprovoked seizures have occurred, the risk of further seizures is 70–80%, justifying the diagnosis of epilepsy. There are no clear data on the risk of multiple further seizures; however it would appear that of all children presenting with a first seizure, only about one in three or 30% will go on to have > ten seizures over the next ten years (15).

Likelihood of remission

The overall likelihood of remission following new-onset epilepsy is approximately 50–60%. In a recent prospective study, 74% of 613 children had remission of seizures on daily medication defined as seizure freedom for two years, although 24% later relapsed with more seizures. About half of the relapses occurred when medication was being withdrawn, while a quarter had relapses while they were still being treated. Idiopathic generalized epilepsy syndromes that have an onset between five and nine years of age are associated with substantially better remission rates. In contrast, remote symptomatic etiology (e.g., cerebral dysgenesis or as a sequel to severe peri-natal hypoxic–ischemic encephalopathy or meningitis), a family history of epilepsy, higher seizure frequency and slow-wave activity on the initial EEG are risk factors associated with a reduced likelihood of achieving remission. Young age of onset (less than one year of age) and seizure type were not important risk factors for achieving seizure control (16).

In general, the specific epilepsy syndrome remains important in predicting the likelihood of remission, although few epilepsy syndromes have a 'guaranteed' good or bad prognosis. In general, we estimate that 75% of children with epilepsy have a syndrome with an 'in between' prognosis – some remit and others do not. Children with benign epilepsy with centro-temporal spikes (benign rolandic epilepsy) always remit by mid-adolescence as do those with early-onset benign occipital epilepsy and benign myoclonic epilepsy of infancy. Lennox–Gastaut syndrome, Dravet syndrome (severe myoclonic epilepsy of infancy) and Sturge–Weber and Rasmussen's syndromes will almost never remit spontaneously. Many syndromes are unlikely to remit although there are a number of exceptions. For example, children who experienced West syndrome in the first year of life may show early remission, but in the long term 60–75% will continue to have seizures, while 25–40% will remain seizure-free.

Additional syndromes that are often drug resistant include symptomatic focal epilepsies caused by hippocampal sclerosis, malformations of cortical development and other cerebral pathology. Juvenile myoclonic epilepsy may eventually remit but most patients (approximately 80%) will require long-term antiepileptic treatment.

A precise and accurate prediction of remission for children with epilepsy remains elusive. A study of over 1,000 children with epilepsy followed for at least five years concluded that comprehensive statistical models make the wrong prediction in 30% of cases; some predicted to remit do not, and vice versa (17).

Recurrence risk after AED withdrawal

Up to 70% of children with epilepsy respond to antiepileptic therapy and will enter early and prolonged seizure remission shortly after starting treatment. For these children it is important to balance seizure freedom, the likelihood of spontaneous remission and side effects of long-term AED treatment (e.g., on mood, behavior, memory, libido, fertility, contraception and pregnancy). As epilepsy is not a single disorder, average risks for seizure relapse after drug withdrawal may not be relevant to an individual patient. All epilepsy syndromes require an individualized approach. This is well illustrated by adolescents with juvenile myoclonic epilepsy, who have a very high relapse risk for myoclonic and tonic-clonic seizures after drug cessation, whereas nearly all children with benign rolandic epilepsy will remit permanently with or without antiepileptic medication.

A number of factors have been reported to be associated with a greater risk of relapse including a symptomatic cause, an adolescent-onset, rather than a childhood-onset of seizures and an abnormal EEG prior to withdrawal (18, 19).

The Medical Research Council (MRC) Antiepileptic Drug Withdrawal Study Group undertook a large prospective randomized trial in an attempt to provide a more individual prediction of risk of recurrence (20). Most patients were adults and had been seizure-free for two years. One group continued on AED treatment and the other discontinued medication. Twenty two percent of patients who continued medication had a seizure recurrence compared to 41% who were randomized to stop treatment slowly. A Cox proportional hazards model identified several factors that increased the risk of seizure recurrence including:

- being 16 years or older at the diagnosis of epilepsy
- taking more than one antiepileptic drug
- experiencing seizures after starting antiepileptic drug treatment
- a history of primary or secondary generalized tonic-clonic seizures
- a history of myoclonic seizures
- an abnormal EEG.

The risks of seizures recurring decreased with increasing time without seizures, a largely predictable finding. A complex statistical model was developed to allow an estimation of the risk of seizures recurring in the next one and two years with either continued antiepileptic drug treatment or slow withdrawal of medication. Unfortunately, the study did not include many children and it is therefore unclear if this somewhat complicated predictive model is valid for a pediatric population.

There are currently no comprehensive data to substantiate the risks associated with a rapid or slow rate of withdrawal of AEDs. One pediatric study showed no difference in seizure relapse rate following a rapid (average six weeks) or slow (average nine months) taper of medication (21). The rate of drug withdrawal is likely only to have an effect on the incidence of acute withdrawal seizures, and not on the natural history of the epilepsy and whether it is likely to relapse.

Risk of refractory epilepsy

If seizures are not controlled after treatment with two optimal regimens of AEDs, seizure remission may still nevertheless occur, eventually. However, many will continue to have seizures and a referral to a tertiary care epilepsy center is necessary for more 'aggressive' and alternative therapies, and specifically for possible surgical evaluation (22).

Risks of status epilepticus

Convulsive status epilepticus (CSE) constitutes a neurologic emergency, which frequently occurs in the context of an acute provocation (e.g., fever, meningitis, encephalitis) but also commonly occurs in patients who already have an established diagnosis of epilepsy. The incidence is highest in children, particularly infants, and the elderly. The risk for CSE has been estimated at approximately 10% to 20% in a Finnish study in children following the initial diagnosis of epilepsy. The highest risk for CSE appears to be early in the course of epilepsy and almost all CSE in children will occur at onset or within two years of initial diagnosis (23). Prolonged seizures have a clear tendency to repeat themselves and a prior history of CSE is a substantial risk factor for recurrent episodes of CSE. Approximately one-third of children who have already suffered from CSE will experience at least one further episode. Further independent, but intercorrelated risk factors for CSE include:
- a young age of onset (less than three years of age)
- a symptomatic etiology (i.e., a known or identified cause)
- the diagnosis of an epileptic encephalopathy.

The underlying etiology of CSE usually dictates the risk for neurologic sequelae and mortality. Convulsive status epilepticus poses a severe risk for mortality only in the context of a severe neurologic insult. Mortality directly related to the episode of convulsive status epilepticus itself appears low (0–2%); it remains higher in acute symptomatic convulsive status epilepticus (12.5–16%) and particularly in acute central nervous system infections (24).

Status epilepticus that presents as the first seizure (before the diagnosis of epilepsy) is associated with an increased risk of death. This again is related to the underlying etiology, including a severe infection of the central nervous system or a neuro-degenerative disorder (25). Fortunately, patients who present with *de novo* CSE appear to have a low risk (<10%) of neuro-developmental sequelae (24).

The prompt use of benzodiazepines in the treatment of CSE appears to have dramatically reduced the incidence of the syndrome termed 'hemiconvulsion, hemiplegia and epilepsy' (HHE), a disorder when a severe focal status epilepticus is followed by permanent and unilateral brain damage. Consequently, parents of children with epilepsy should be counseled about the risks for CSE, and appropriate and early treatment measures need to be instituted if seizures do not terminate spontaneously. The use of rectal diazepam or buccal or nasal midazolam in the community (home and school/college) is appropriate for children at high risk for developing CSE; these include children with a young age of onset of their epilepsy, a symptomatic etiology, an epileptic encephalopathy or a prior episode of CSE.

Minimizing risks

First aid for seizures

First aid for seizures aims to protect and prevent the child and adolescent from harm and injury during a seizure. Many people have little understanding of how to respond to a seizure. Guidelines for seizure first aid are readily available from the Epilepsy Foundation of America and UK-based epilepsy charities (Epilepsy Action, the National Society for Epilepsy, and the National Centre for Young People with Epilepsy). The main goal of seizure first aid is to protect the person from injury caused by a change of awareness or loss of consciousness during a complex partial seizure or a generalized tonic-clonic seizure. The majority of seizures (including tonic-clonic seizures) last less than three minutes and are self-limiting, but if a seizure continues longer than five minutes it is usually appropriate to initiate appropriate emergency care.

Key points have been provided (www.epilepsyfoundation.org and www.epilepsy.org.uk) on how to respond to persons who are having a seizure. If the seizure is focal or complex partial then it is appropriate to watch the person closely but allow them to wander safely and guide them away from danger. Remaining calm and reassuring and staying with the person until awareness has returned is self-evident. If the seizure is a convulsion, first aid basics start with the ability to recognize the tonic-clonic seizure (several graphic illustrations are provided), again to remain calm, to attempt to lower the person gently to the ground, cushion the head, loosen clothing around the neck, turn the person on their side to keep the airway clear (termed the 'recovery position'). Physical restraint, placing objects into the mouth or giving the person medications by mouth or something to drink are all contra-indicated. Documenting the duration and manifestation of the seizure is helpful and again it is mandatory to stay with the person until the seizure is over (26). This is because the person may be confused following the seizure, will not appreciate what has happened to them and may behave inappropriately or even aggressively; this may be misinterpreted as representing alcohol- or drug-induced behavior with obvious consequences.

Treatment protocols to minimize risks for children with prolonged seizures and status epilepticus

The risk of prolonged seizures (defined arbitrarily as a seizure lasting between five minutes and 30 minutes) and status epilepticus (defined as a seizure lasting longer than 30 minutes) can be reduced through appropriate, prompt and aggressive interventions outside the hospital, where most episodes begin. Evidence suggests that early intervention reduces the likelihood of a seizure lasting longer than 60 minutes (27). Interventions should not wait for 30 minutes; if the seizure lasts five minutes or longer, it is time to respond. Interventions can be implemented at home, in daycare and school settings. A useful plan should be initiated at five minutes rather than 30 minutes and be taught to the child's care-givers including the family, and child-minders/baby-sitters, school personnel, and emergency medical services. Most intervention plans include home administration of a benzodiazepine. Most studies have investigated rectal diazepam (0.5 mg/kg) but randomized trials suggested that buccal midazolam (0.2 mg/kg) (28) or 0.5 mg/kg (29) is more effective.

We believe that all care-givers should be taught formally by qualified medical personnel about when precisely and how much benzodiazepine to give because excessive doses of benzodiazepines may cause respiratory depression. The intervention plan should be individualized and written in simple language that takes into account the sophistication of the family and other care-givers and the proximity to a hospital. The emergency intervention should include 'rules' for calling emergency medical services; for many patients it is not necessary to go to a hospital if the seizure stops after a dose of benzodiazepine. If the child is transferred to hospital established protocols for treatment of status are available (30, 31). This is discussed in more detail in Chapter 6.

Risks of antiepileptic drugs

The selection of an antiepileptic drug should obviously be undertaken in partnership with the family, and usually be based on the epilepsy syndrome, the safety profile of the drug and with an appropriate formulation for the child. Ease of dosing and titration and tolerability are important factors. The severity of the seizures needs to be balanced with the risk of side effects of the medications. No AED is free from adverse effects but some have a higher risk than others. Newer AEDs are reportedly better tolerated than the older agents although, particularly in children, there are few large randomized trials to confirm this impression.

The mechanisms of action of many AEDs are uncertain but in some way most block seizure propagation by reducing neuronal hyperexcitability through altering membrane excitability, increasing post-synaptic inhibition or modifying the synchronization of neuronal networks. Not surprisingly, these effects may also interfere with normal central nervous system functions at therapeutic doses, which lead to the common short-term predictable side effects including dizziness and drowsiness and possible mood changes. Side effects may be dose-dependent and predictable or idiosyncratic and unpredictable; some AEDs may show both idiosyncratic and dose-dependent side effects.

Dose-related side effects

Dose-related side effects are typically directly related to the pharmacological effects of the AED and are mostly mild and alleviated by dose reduction. Central nervous system side effects such as dizziness may be seen at initiation of the drug following which there may be functional tolerance. Dose reduction and a slower titration rate may eliminate the problem.

Dose-related side effects may rarely be more dangerous. A rash is a relatively common side effect that may be mild and transient, but occasionally serious and life-threatening. A rash is usually unpredictable and therefore idiosyncratic; however, for several drugs it appears to be more common with rapid introduction and in that sense is dose-dependent. A rash is particularly likely to occur with the use of lamotrigine, carbamazepine, phenytoin and phenobarbital. It is usually seen in the first six weeks following the drug's introduction and is a reason to discontinue the medication immediately. In its most severe form it may rapidly develop into Stevens–Johnson syndrome. This is particularly likely with lamotrigine and in young children the frequency has been reported to be between 1 in 50 and 1 in 300 (32). Fortunately the incidence of Stevens–Johnson decreased markedly with a recommendation for slower dose titration over many weeks or a few months. Carbamazepine, oxcarbazepine, phenytoin and phenobarbital share a similar chemical structure with the potential for cross-reactivity. A child with a severe rash from one of these three drugs should generally be treated next with a drug with a very different chemical structure. However, it may be appropriate to use oxcarbazepine (cautiously) in children who previously had experienced a rash with carbamazepine as there may be reduced cross-reactivity,

Idiosyncratic reactions

Idiosyncratic reactions cannot be predicted based on the pharmacologic properties of the drug, are individual-dependent and can be serious and life-threatening. They may be acute, occurring soon after therapy is commenced, or chronic, occurring after many years. They may also affect any body system. Since most of these reactions are uncommon they are often not defined in the pre-marketing phase of drug development.

Hematological abnormalities are associated with several AEDs:
- aplastic anemia with felbamate and carbamazepine
- agranulocytosis with carbamazepine and phenytoin
- thrombocytopenia with valproic acid.

The overall risk of blood dyscrasias in one cohort taking carbamazepine, phenytoin, phenobarbital or sodium valproate was estimated to be 3–4/100,000 prescriptions (33). Liver toxicity has been observed with many AEDs. Sodium valproate may be associated with dose-related mild elevations of transaminases in about 40% but this does not indicate toxicity. The risk of liver failure is highest among children under two years of age on polytherapy (1 in 500 to 1 in 8,000 in older children); however, it is suspected that many of the children in this age range diagnosed with valproate-induced liver failure have Alpers' disease, which is a neuro-degenerative disorder that includes liver failure even if there has been no exposure to valproic acid (sodium valproate) (34). Other children who show liver dysfunction probably have another mitochondrial or other metabolic disorder that may be exacerbated by this AED. It is therefore suggested that sodium valproate be used with caution in children aged three years (and under) and in whom the underlying etiology of the epilepsy is unclear. Felbamate was also associated with an increased risk of liver failure, estimated at 1 per 18,500–25,000 exposures.

An unusual but important side effect of another AED, vigabatrin, is visual field constriction that may affect up to 40% of adults (probably less frequently in children) and usually in high doses. In adults, the visual field deficit has been reported, rarely, to develop as early as one to six months after the start of treatment; far more frequently it may develop after one or two years. It may also be related to the daily dose. It is difficult to assess the incidence of the visual field deficit in children (particularly in those with cognitive dysfunction) because a formal and reliable visual field-testing demands a cognitive age of at least nine or ten years of age. Vigabatrin remains a first-line medication for infantile spasms, especially when the cause is tuberous sclerosis. As short a course of vigabatrin as possible, possibly four to six months, seems wise in these children, as the response rate is both rapid (often within five to ten days) and sustained. Based on current information, it is very unlikely that any visual field deficit will develop following this short treatment period. Obviously, visual fields cannot be assessed in these children because of their age and usual cognitive difficulties.

Long-term risk of antiepileptic drugs

There are limited data about other long-term risks of AEDs. Gingival hyperplasia and facial coarsening often complicate long-term, high-dose treatment with phenytoin. Vitamin D status and bone health remain a concern for individuals receiving AEDs, particularly, but not only, those drugs that induce the cytochrome P450 enzyme system. Compounding factors include neurological disability with decreased weight-bearing and decreased exposure to sunshine. The role of monitoring with dual energy x-ray absorptiometry (DEXA) scans in children remains unclear. The current recommendation is that most children who are treated with long-term AEDs should receive supplemental calcium and vitamin D, although it is unclear how effective this will be in reducing the risk and incidence of fractures. In addition, this recommendation is unlikely to be followed in practice.

Effects of AEDs on the unborn fetus

Pre-natal exposure to AEDs increases the risk of both minor and major congenital malformations. This is particularly likely with phenytoin, phenobarbital and valproic acid; children exposed to valproic acid during pregnancy may also show cognitive problems, especially communication and language dysfunction. Counseling about this risk is important if girls with epilepsy are at all likely to continue AEDs beyond puberty, particularly because a high proportion of pregnancies are unplanned. In addition, many AEDs interfere with the effectiveness of oral contraceptives (particularly, phenobarbital, phenytoin, carbamazepine, oxcarbazepine, topiramate and high-dose lamotrigine). The major malformation rate in all AED-exposed pregnancies is 3.5–9%, compared to a background risk of 1–2% with a higher risk observed in those exposed to polytherapy, and particularly if valproate or phenytoin are part of the polytherapy (35). Avoiding these risks to the fetus is not simple. Preconceptual folate has not been shown to be effective in reducing the incidence of major or minor malformations, but may be worthwhile, in a daily dose of 5 mg. Reducing or stopping AEDs prior to pregnancy will lower the threshold for tonic-clonic seizures, which may be very harmful to the fetus and the woman, and may potentially result in fetal or maternal death, or both.

The relative risks of individual AEDs are becoming apparent from prospective pregnancy registries and there does not appear to be a completely safe agent; predictably there are more data on the older than newer AEDs. We recommend that this issue be discussed with younger adolescents, including careful discussion of appropriate contraception and a plea for both planned pregnancies and pregnancies that are preceded by consultation with a well-informed and interested clinician or, ideally, by a joint consultation with a neurologist and obstetrician.

Cognitive and behavioral effects

Cognitive, psychiatric and behavioral side effects of AEDs have been extensively reported in children with epilepsy. The effect of a specific AED in an individual patient may be difficult to assess because cognitive, psychiatric and behavioral problems are prevalent in a number of children with epilepsy at the time of diagnosis and before treatment. Although there are striking individual exceptions, in general the risks for behavioral and psychiatric side effects are less in patients who receive AED monotherapy, have good seizure control and have no other neurological dysfunction. Higher rates of negative behavior and depression have been noted with AEDs that have a strong GABA-ergic mechanism of action (e.g., phenobarbital, benzodiazepines); however, topiramate and, to a lesser extent, levetiracetam do not significantly interact with GABA transmission but may still be associated with severe behavior problems, including depression and suicidal ideation. Some AEDs are noted for improved mood and are used widely for psychiatric indications including carbamazepine, lamotrigine and valproic acid. Nearly all AEDs have occasionally induced a catastrophic behavioral deterioriation including acute psychosis with delusions, mood changes, hypomania and mania, anxiety with depersonalization or even conversion reactions. This type of reaction has been particularly problematic with phenobarbital, which limits it use, but also with gabapentin, topiramate and vigabatrin.

It is unclear if pre-existing behavioral problems increase the risk for AED-induced problems; however adolescents with psychiatric co-morbidities may have an increased suicide risk when an AED that induces CP450 reduces the effect of their antidepressant medications. Inhibitors of CP450 such as valproic acid may result in toxic levels of anxiolytics including diazepam or alprazolam. These types of interactions may be minimized by the use of non-enzyme inducing AEDs including gabapentin, oxcarbazepine, levetiracetam or lacosamide (36).

Cognitive side effects of AEDs may be difficult to assess, particularly if the child has significant pre-existing cognitive difficulties (mental handicap). Topiramate is probably associated with the most frequent and severe cognitive difficulties, including language (word-finding) and memory impairment.

These many factors will impact on the choice and dosage regimen of AEDs. There are no simple, validated, clinic-friendly screening tests to detect behavioral, psychiatric and cognitive side effects. Before the prescription of an AED, the clinician should discuss these issues with the family (and whenever appropriate, the child), and then reconsider them shortly after starting treatment. The opinion of teachers and other professionals who know the child well can be very helpful but if there is doubt about significant changes in behavior or cognition, or both, then it may be appropriate to prescribe an alternate AED with a different mechanism of action. Several years of adverse effects may potentially affect the child's life forever.

Risk of weight gain and obesity in children with epilepsy

The risk of obesity among children with epilepsy is multifactorial and may be attributed to increased appetite induced by some AEDs (particularly valproic acid), reduced physical activity as the result of restrictions, some of which may be inappropriate, neuro-endocrine dysfunction including polycystic ovary syndrome and epilepsy-mediated dysfunction. Other factors may also contribute to the obesity, including physical and mental disabilities, depression and anxiety disorders.

Obesity has recently also been reported as a common co-morbidity for pediatric patients with untreated, newly diagnosed epilepsy (37). In this study, almost 39% of 251 children with newly diagnosed untreated epilepsy were overweight or obese (as defined by a body mass index [BMI] $\geq$ 85th percentile for age). Using adjusted BMI Z-scores, differences in age, etiology and concomitant non-epilepsy medications were significant factors. Adolescents had higher adjusted BMI Z-scores than younger patients; patients with symptomatic epilepsy had lower BMI Z-scores than patients with idiopathic epilepsy, as did patients on stimulant psychotropic medication compared to those on no medication. In summary, obesity does appear to be a common and probably under-appreciated co-morbid problem in children with newly diagnosed and untreated epilepsy. It also appears to be correlated with increasing age, idiopathic etiology and absence of concomitant medication (37).

Psychosocial risks and hazards of childhood epilepsy

Quality of life

While the first goal in treatment for children with epilepsy is to establish seizure freedom without AED side effects, there is an increasing recognition that children with epilepsy are at significant risk of poor quality of life during childhood and on into adult life. Health-related quality of life refers to a child's and/or the care-giver's perception of the child's state of functioning and well-being across multiple areas or domains. These commonly include physical, psychological and social functioning and an overall sense of well-being. For some scales, specific issues related to epilepsy are also included. The domains are likely to differ from child to child and family to family; what may be important for one child/family may be far less important for another child/family.

The following five quality-of-life domains appear to be most relevant for children with epilepsy (38):

- epilepsy and treatment: neurologic, physical and cognitive functioning, seizure, epilepsy syndrome and antiepileptic drug-related effects
- psychological: mood, behavioral dysfunction, anxiety, depression, psychiatric diagnoses, self-esteem and perception of having epilepsy
- social: peer and family relationships, restrictions, isolation and engagement in activities
- school: academic achievement, learning problems, adaptive behavior and attitudes
- family: psychological adjustment, seizure management and general coping skills, support, attitude, concerns and fears, perception of stigma, leisure activities.

Children with epilepsy have been found to have poorer functioning and a reduced sense of well-being in the psychological, social and school domains of quality of life when compared with children with asthma, even when the epilepsy was inactive (39). Difficulties in the social domain were related to the severity of the epilepsy. Girls had more difficulty in the psychological domain, including demonstrating more anxiety and more negative feelings about having epilepsy than boys. Concerns in children appear to focus primarily around medication and seizure issues in contrast to parental concerns which seem to focus on their child's future, their seizures and their school performance. To date there are no interventions that have been proven to improve quality of life in children with epilepsy.

Psychological risks of epilepsy

Children with epilepsy are about five times more likely to have mental health concerns than children without epilepsy (40). The risks for mental health dysfunction are mainly in the areas of internalizing behavior such as anxiety and depression, attention deficit and somatic complaints. The extent of psychological problems seen in children with epilepsy is much higher than in children with other chronic disorders. Specifically, the prevalence of psychiatric disorders is over twice as common as in children with diabetes, suggesting that the generic effect of chronic illness is amplified in epilepsy by other factors including neuro-biological (e.g., medications, neuro-endocrine, neurotransmitter abnormalities, neurological deficits), individual resilience and societal factors in dealing with the specific stresses of being faced with unpredictable seizures (40). There is little information on the coping responses and perceptions of children with epilepsy but one study suggested that those with a sense of competence and optimism, a willingness to seek support and compliant style have fewer behavioral problems and a better concept of 'self.' Those with more behavior problems and lower self-esteem are more likely to 'feel different' than others and be more irritable (including aggressive) and socially withdrawn. Negative attitudes are related to poorer self-esteem and behavior problems and to low satisfaction with family relationships and an 'unknown' locus of control (41).

It is interesting that approximately one-third of children with newly diagnosed epilepsy already have behavior problems, indicating that seizures themselves are only one factor responsible for the high rate of psychiatric disorders in epilepsy (42). Early and ongoing psychological assessments and support may be needed to minimize the risk of developing mental health problems in this vulnerable patient population.

School-functioning

Children with epilepsy have frequent cognitive deficits before the diagnosis. Not surprisingly, academic performance is often suboptimal. In addition, those with refractory epilepsy may have seizure-related intermittent difficulties with memory, fatigue and a discontinuous learning experience owing to the seizures, frequent hospitalizations and school absenteeism. Problems in school may also affect other aspects of the child's behaviour and emotional well-being, including motivation, self-esteem and peer relationships, and may consequently lead to potentially spiraling mental health problems.

Family

A family's adjustment to their child's epilepsy and their psychological functioning are important and closely linked. A chronic condition such as epilepsy may negatively affect the adjustment of other family members, especially the mother (36). The parents' ability to manage the epilepsy and adjust psychologically will allow them to exert the most positive influence on their child's quality of life and minimize the risks of the psychosocial burden of the epilepsy on their child. Understanding the family's dynamics and interactions, and cohesiveness will be important for appropriate support and intervention from professionals to reduce the risk of the epilepsy burden on the family. Check the following:
- are there undue and unnecessary restrictions of leisure activity on all family members because of the epilepsy?
- is parental supervision of the child's activities appropriate?
- are parental concerns about the stigma of epilepsy appropriate or exaggerated?
- are there excessive fears regarding the child's condition?
- is there a healthy sense of competency in dealing with seizures?

Impact of intractable epilepsy as perceived by children and adolescents

A recent qualitative study of children and adolescents with medically refractory epilepsy undergoing surgical evaluation explored the 'intrusive' role of seizures on various aspects of the youths' lives (43). They were at risk for excessive fatigue and inertia and multiple somatic symptoms because of their antiepileptic drugs including headaches, hair loss, sore mouth from seizures, visual disturbances, clumsiness, increased appetite, weight gain and dizziness. In addition there was an intermittent heightening of emotional suffering with adolescents, reporting periods of intense emotional distress that they attributed mainly to the unpredictability of seizures and physical loss of control during a seizure. There is also an increased risk of suffering multiple emotions including worry, fear, panic, anger, pain, frustration, embarrassment, sadness and depression. In the social domain, a profound sense of social isolation was a dominant theme in the interviews conducted with adolescents in this study. The risk of social isolation was closely related to a lack of self-confidence, exclusionary behavior (barriers) by peers and excessive parental monitoring and limit-setting. Other studies have suggested that the perception of being different from their peers is also an important factor and contributes to irregular compliance (concordance) with taking their antiepileptic medication and clinic attendance.

Long-term outcome and impact of childhood-onset epilepsy into adulthood

Only a few studies have documented the social outcome of adults with childhood-onset epilepsy. Approximately 30% of children who develop epilepsy have concomitant learning difficulties, which may be moderate to severe in degree. It is not easy to define what constitutes a good social outcome for this group although one population-based study did document very high rates of social dependency but without social isolation (9). A number of studies from Finland have tracked the life experiences for 100 patients with childhood-onset epilepsy and 'epilepsy only' – (i.e., they had no additional co-morbid significant neurological deficits or mental retardation). When assessed 30–35 years after seizure onset and compared with controls, those still requiring AED treatment did not function as well in adult life when compared with those whose epilepsy had remitted (44, 45). Those who remained on medication, and irrespective of seizure control, showed higher rates of unemployment and lower socioeconomic status than controls. However, all adults with childhood-onset epilepsy, regardless of remission or medication status, were more likely to have educational failure, and less likely to be married and have children.

A population-based study from Nova Scotia of children with epilepsy recorded their social outcome 10–30 years later (44). Even those with apparent 'normal' intelligence showed high rates of:

- academic failure
- unemployment
- social isolation
- inadvertent, unplanned pregnancy
- psychiatric care.

Remission of epilepsy (defined as being seizure-free and off AED treatment) did not predict social outcome (46). Even patients with childhood absence epilepsy showed high rates of social problems as young adults (47).

For many children with epilepsy, their social outcome as adults will be unsatisfactory, even in the 50% whose epilepsy remits. Close and sustained attention to educational and sexuality issues seems wise if not important when caring for children with epilepsy, despite the fact that no intervention has been shown to improve long-term social outcome.

Perception of risk and prevention

It is frequently a challenging task to assist families to come to terms with and understand the risks and hazards faced by their children with epilepsy. The subjective interpretation of risk may be driven by personal experiences, social–cultural background and beliefs, the resources and abilities to control a particular risk, the exposure to education and knowledge on the topic of risk.

Misconceptions persist, as do indifferences and complacencies over risks in the day-to-day world of the child with epilepsy and the family. As clinicians, and with other involved professionals, we can, and should, actively address these issues. This includes being both interested and appropriately trained in the diagnosis and management of epilepsy, but also in adopting a truly holistic approach. This must include a more integrated management model that should not avoid but address and discuss the real risks and hazards of childhood epilepsy and in an appropriate, realistic and non-alarmist way.

REFERENCES

1. Brnich MJ, Mallett LG. Focus on prevention: conducting a hazard risk assessment. U.S. Department of Health and Human services, Public Health Service, Centers for Disease Control and Prevention, National Institute for Occupational Safety and Health, July 2003.
2. Beghi E. Accidents and injuries in patients with epilepsy. *Expert Rev Neurother* 2009; **9**: 291–8.
3. Beghi E, Brown S, Capurro D, *et al.* IBE Commission Report. 2nd Workshop on 'Epilepsy, Risks, and Insurance'. *Epilepsia* 2000; **41**: 110–12.
4. Wirrell EC, Camfield PR, Camfield CS, Dooley JM, Gordon KE. Accidental injury is a serious risk in children with typical absence epilepsy. *Arch Neurol* 1996; **53**: 929–32.
5. Kemp AM, Sibert JR. Epilepsy in children and the risk of drowning. *Arch Dis Child* 1993; **68**: 684–5.
6. Orlowski JP, Rothner AD, Lueders H. Submersion accidents in children with epilepsy. *Am J Dis Child* 1982; **136**: 777–80.
7. Camfield CS, Camfield PR, Veugelers PJ. Death in children with epilepsy: a population-based study. *Lancet* 2002; **359**: 1891–5.
8. Callenbach PM, Westendorp RG, Geerts AT, *et al.* Mortality risk in children with epilepsy: the Dutch study of epilepsy in childhood. *Pediatrics* 2001; **107**: 1259–63.
9. Camfield C, Camfield P. Twenty years after childhood-onset symptomatic generalized epilepsy the social outcome is usually dependency or death: a population-based study. *Dev Med Child Neurol* 2008; **50**: 859–63.
10. Tomson T, Nashef L, Ryvlin P. Sudden unexpected death in epilepsy: current knowledge and future directions. *Lancet Neurol* 2008; **7**: 1021–31.
11. Nashef L, Fish DR, Garner S, Sander JW, Shorvon SD. Sudden death in epilepsy: a study of incidence in a young cohort with epilepsy and learning difficulty. *Epilepsia* 1995; **36**: 1187–94.
12. Appleton RE. Mortality in pediatric epilepsy. *Arch Dis Child* 2003; **88**: 1091–4.
13. Gayatri NA, Morrall MC, Jain V, *et al.* Parental and physician beliefs regarding the provision and content of written sudden unexpected death in epilepsy (SUDEP) information. *Epilepsia* 2010; **51**: 777–82.

14. Berg AT, Shinnar S. The risk of seizure recurrence following a first unprovoked seizure: a quantitative review. *Neurology* 1991; **41**: 965–72.

15. Shinnar S, Berg AT, Moshe SL, *et al.* The risk of seizure recurrence after a first unprovoked afebrile seizure in childhood. An extended follow up. *Pediatrics* 1996; **98**: 216–25.

16. Berg AT, Shinnar S, Levy SR, *et al.* Two-year remission and subsequent relapse in children with newly diagnosed epilepsy. *Epilepsia* 2001; **42**: 1553–62.

17. Geelhoed M, Boerrigter AO, Camfield P, *et al.* The accuracy of outcome prediction models for childhood-onset epilepsy. *Epilepsia* 2005; **46**: 1526–32.

18. Berg AT, Shinnar S. Relapse following discontinuation of antiepileptic drugs: a meta-analysis. *Neurology* 1994; **44**: 601–8.

19. Andersson T, *et al.* A comparison between one and three years of treatment in uncomplicated childhood epilepsy: a prospective study. II. The EEG as predictor of outcome after withdrawal of treatment. *Epilepsia* 1997; **38**: 225–32.

20. Prognostic index for recurrence of seizures after remission of epilepsy. Medical Research Council Antiepileptic Drug Withdrawal Study Group. *BMJ* 1993: **306**: 1374–8.

21. Ranganathan LN, Ramaratnam S. Rapid versus slow withdrawal of antiepileptic drugs. *Cochrane Database Syst Rev* 2006: Apr **19** (2): CD005003.

22. Berg AT, Levy SR, Testa FM, D'Souza R. Remission of epilepsy after two drug failures in children: a prospective study. *Ann Neurol* 2009; **65**: 510–19.

23. Sillanpää M, Shinnar S. Status epilepticus in a population-based cohort with childhood-onset epilepsy in Finland. *Ann Neurol* 2002; **52**: 303–10.

24. Raspall-Chaure M, Chin RF, Neville BG, Scott RC. Outcome of pediatric convulsive status epilepticus: a systematic review. *Lancet Neurol* 2006; **5**: 769–79.

25. Berg AT, Shinnar S, Testa FM, *et al.* Status epilepticus after the initial diagnosis of epilepsy in children. *Neurology* 2004; **63**: 1027–34.

26. O'Hara KA. First aid for seizures: the importance of education and appropriate response. *J Child Neurol* 2007; **22** (Suppl 5): S30–37.

27. Chin RF, Verhulst L, Neville BG, Peters MJ, Scott RC. Inappropriate emergency management of status epilepticus in children contributes to need for intensive care. *J Neurol Neurosurg Psychiatry* 2004; **75**: 1584–8.

28. Scott RC, Besag FM, Neville BG. Buccal midazolam and rectal diazepam for treatment of prolonged seizures in childhood and adolescence: a randomised trial. *Lancet* 1999; **353**: 623–6.

29. McIntyre J, Robertson S, Norris E, *et al.* Safety and efficacy of buccal midazolam versus rectal diazepam for emergency treatment of seizures in children: a randomized controlled trial. *Lancet* 2005; **366**: 205–10.

30. Appleton R, Choonara I, Martland T, *et al.* The treatment of convulsive status epilepticus in children. The Status Epilepticus Working Party, Members of the Status Epilepticus Working Party. *Arch Dis Child* 2000; **83**: 415–19.

31. Epilepsy Foundation of America. Treatment of convulsive status epilepticus. Recommendations of the Epilepsy Foundation of America's Working Group on Status Epilepticus. *JAMA* 1993; **270**: 854–9.

32. Perucca E, Beghi E, Dulac O, Shorvon S, Tomson T. Assessing risk-to-benefit ratio in antiepileptic drug therapy. *Epilepsy Res* 2000; **41**: 107–39.

33. Blackburn SC, Oliart AD, Garcia Rodriguez LA, Perez Gutthann S. Antiepileptics and blood dyscrasias: a cohort study. *Pharmacotherapy* 1998; **18**: 1277–83.

34. Dreifuss FE, Langer DH, Moline KA, Maxwell JE. Valproic acid hepatic fatalities. II. US experience since 1984. *Neurology* 1989; **39**: 201–7.

35. Cross JH. Neuro-developmental effects of AEDs. *Epilepsy Res* 2010; **88**: 1–10.

36. Glauser TA. Behavioral and psychiatric adverse events associated with antiepileptic drugs commonly used in pediatric patients. *J Child Neurol* 2004; **19** (Suppl 1): S25–38.
37. Daniels ZS, Nick TG, Liu C, Cassedy A, Glauser TA. Obesity is a common comorbidity for pediatric patients with untreated, newly diagnosed epilepsy. *Neurology* 2009; **73**: 658–64.
38. Austin JK, Caplan R. Behavioral and psychiatric comorbidities in pediatric epilepsy. *Epilepsia* 2007; **48**: 1639–51.
39. Austin JK, Huster GA, Dunn DW, Risinger MW. Adolescents with active or inactive epilepsy or asthma: a comparison of quality of life. *Epilepsia* 1996; **37**: 1228–38.
40. Davies S, Heyman I, Goodman R. A population survey of mental health problems in children with epilepsy. *Dev Med Child Neurol* 2003; **45**: 292–5.
41. Dunn DW, Austin JK, Perkins SM. Prevalence of psychopathology in childhood epilepsy: categorical and dimensional measures. *Dev Med Child Neurol* 2009: **51**: 364–72.
42. Fastenau PS, Johnson CS, Perkins SM, *et al.* Neuropsychologic status at seizure onset in children: risk factors for early cognitive deficits. *Neurology* 2009; **73**: 526–34.
43. Elliott IM, Lach L, Smith ML. I just want to be normal: a qualitative study exploring how children and adolescents view the impact of intractable epilepsy on their quality of life. *Epilepsy Behav* 2005; **7**: 664–78.
44. Sillanpää M, Haataja L, Shinnar S. Perceived impact of childhood-onset epilepsy on quality of life as an adult. *Epilepsia* 2004; **45**: 971–7.
45. Jalaya M, Sillanpää M, Camfield C, Camfield P. Social adjustment and competence 35 years after onset of childhood epilepsy: a prospective controlled study. *Epilepsia* 1997; **38**: 708–15.
46. Camfield CS, Camfield PR. Long-term social outcomes for children with epilepsy. *Epilepsia* 2007; **48** (Suppl 9): S3–5.
47. Wirrell EC, Camfield CS, Camfield PR, *et al.* Long-term psychosocial outcome in typical absence epilepsy. Sometimes a wolf in sheep's clothing. *Arch Pediatr Adolesc Med* 1997; **151**: 152–8.

6

Status epilepticus

Richard Appleton and Peter Camfield

Convulsive status epilepticus

Convulsive status epilepticus (CSE), whether febrile or afebrile, is a medical emergency and is associated with a significant morbidity, including mortality. Although the morbidity of CSE is predominantly related to the age of the child, its etiology and duration, it is also clearly related to its management. Both the under- and over-treatment of CSE may result in irreversible consequences and, rarely, death.

The majority of tonic-clonic convulsions last three minutes or less; conversely, convulsions that last for five minutes are unlikely to stop spontaneously. In addition, the longer a convulsion lasts, the more difficult it will be to terminate with emergency medication. For this reason, and even though CSE is defined as a convulsion that lasts for 30 minutes or more, in practice, emergency (also called 'rescue') medication will usually be initiated after five minutes.

The initial treatment of a tonic-clonic convulsion is nearly always with a benzodiazepine. Convulsions that occur out of hospital and in the home or school will usually be treated with buccal midazolam or rectal diazepam, or, rarely in the UK, rectal paraldehyde for those children who do not respond to, or develop respiratory suppression with, a benzodiazepine. Most paramedic and ambulance personnel will use rectal diazepam rather than buccal midazolam. Ongoing seizures will then be managed in a hospital Accident and Emergency Department (UK) or Emergency Room (Canada and the USA). On admission, the child's initial management must begin with securing the **a**irway, **b**reathing and **c**irculation, giving high-flow oxygen and measuring a finger-prick blood glucose. For obvious reasons it is important to ensure that the child is experiencing a genuine tonic-clonic seizure and not

Childhood Epilepsy: Management from Diagnosis to Remission, ed. Richard Appleton and Peter Camfield. Published by Cambridge University Press. © Cambridge University Press 2011.

Time	Seizure starts	
0 mins	Check ABC, high-flow O_2 if available Check blood glucose	Confirm clinically that it is an epileptic seizure
5 mins	Midazolam 0.5 mg/kg buccally or Lorazepam 0.1 mg/kg if IV access established	Midazolam may be given by parents, carers or ambulance crew in non-hospital setting
15 mins	Lorazepam 0.1 mg/kg IV	This step should be in hospital Call for senior help Start to prepare phenytoin for step three Re-confirm it is an epileptic seizure
25 mins	Phenytoin 20 mg/kg IV over 20–30 mins **OR** (if on regular phenytoin) Phenobarbital 20 mg/kg IV over 10–20 mins	Paraldehyde 0.8 ml/kg of mixture may be given <u>at the same time as phenytoin</u> as directed by senior medical staff Inform Intensive Care Unit and/or senior anesthetist
45 mins	Rapid sequence induction of anesthesia using thiopentone 4 mg/kg IV	Transfer to PICU

Figure 6.1 Practice parameter for the treatment of convulsive status epilepticus (UK).

a psychogenic, non-epileptic seizure; this is far more commonly seen in adult practice.

Different protocols or algorithms are available and the ones that are currently in use in the UK and Canada are shown in Figures 6.1 and 6.2 respectively. Most, but not all of the components of these protocols are evidence-based, although some of the evidence is very limited. In the USA, fosphenytoin tends to be used in preference to phenytoin because it is associated with a reduced risk of hypotension, cardiac arrhythmias and serious consequences of extravasation (the 'purple hand/glove syndrome'). Fosphenytoin is not used in Canada and the UK not only because of its cost (approximately six times as expensive as phenytoin) but also the potential for over-dosage because it is prescribed as 'phenytoin equivalents.' It is possible that in the future, phenytoin and fosphenytoin may be replaced by intravenous levetiracetam or sodium valproate (valproic acid). A randomized controlled trial is long overdue in which the established anticonvulsant, phenytoin, should be compared against both levetiracetam and sodium valproate (valproic acid).

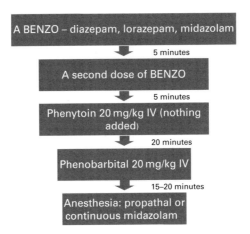

Figure 6.2 Practice parameter for the treatment of convulsive status epilepticus (Canada).

Two crucial issues must be addressed, whichever protocol is used:
a) the specific anticonvulsant must be given in the recommended dose
b) the precise timings of each stage of the protocol (when to 'move on' to the next anticonvulsant in the protocol or algorithm) must be adhered to because the longer the duration of the convulsion or established CSE, the greater the risk of secondary metabolic and hemodynamic consequences, and potentially irreversible sequelae.

Over 56 consultant-years of experience in pediatric epilepsy, supported by recently published community-based studies, have convinced us that children who present in CSE are frequently not appropriately managed according to nationally agreed protocols.

A significant minority of children with CSE will not respond to the treatment protocols and will then be classified as having refractory convulsive status epilepticus (RCSE). All of these children will require immediate discussion with a pediatric intensivist or anesthetist and stabilization. Most will subsequently require admission to an intensive care (therapy) unit and treatment with either thiopentone or a continuous infusion of midazolam. Propofol, commonly used in treating RCSE in adults, is rarely used in children because of its association with profound cardiac dysfunction and metabolic acidosis, which may result in death. The subsequent management of these children is clearly beyond the scope of this chapter.

Non-convulsive status epilepticus

Although non-convulsive status epilepticus (NCSE) is not a medical emergency as in CSE, it is still important to both diagnose and treat. Although NCSE will not result in death, it may be associated with irreversible cognitive and memory dysfunction. The classification of NCSE can be pragmatically outlined as follows:
- absence status (typical, as seen in the idiopathic generalized epilepsies, or atypical, as seen in Lennox–Gastaut syndrome and many of the genetically determined epilepsies, and other symptomatic generalized epilepsy syndromes)

- focal or complex partial status
- continuous spike-wave of slow-sleep (CSWSS): the Landau–Kleffner syndrome (LKS) is a fascinating but rare syndrome that shares some EEG features with CSWSS. Arguably, LKS would more reasonably be included as one of the 'epileptic encephalopathies,' a concept that has been discussed in earlier chapters, rather than a form of NCSE
- hypsarrhythmia (it remains debatable as to whether this could, and should, be included as a form of NCSE, or more appropriately a type of epileptic encephalopathy. Hypsarrhythmia has been discussed in detail in an earlier chapter).

Most children who experience episodes of NCSE will have a symptomatic generalized or focal epilepsy including myoclonic–astatic epilepsy, Lennox–Gastaut syndrome, severe myoclonic epilepsy of infancy (Dravet syndrome) or a specific genetic disorder (e.g., Angelman or Rett syndrome or ring chromosome 20). The diagnosis of NCSE in these children may be difficult because of pre-existing learning or behavior problems, and may be manifest in a number of ways:

- reduced activity, hypotonia or lethargy
- ataxia or tremulousness
- dysarthria, dysphasia or, uncommonly, mutism
- an inability to eat or drink
- altered consciousness ranging from drowsiness through confusion to stupor
- excessive salivation

Typical absence NCSE occurs infrequently in children with an 'idiopathic' generalized epilepsy (childhood-onset or juvenile-onset absence epilepsy). As well as occurring spontaneously in these syndromes, it may also be precipitated by the use of inappropriate antiepileptic drugs (AEDs), and specifically carbamazepine, oxcarbazepine, phenytoin or vigabatrin.

It is important to understand that NCSE may be over-diagnosed, or at least over-considered, in children with learning difficulties or behavioral problems, or both. In some of these situations, the differential diagnosis may include:

- a prolonged post-ictal confusional state
- a side effect of an antiepileptic drug
- substance abuse
- an organic encephalopathy (e.g., caused by hypoglycemia, hypocalcemia) or hydrocephalus
- a dementing disorder (e.g., Huntington's disease, a mitochondrial cytopathy)
- an acute psychosis (specifically a disintegrative psychosis)

The child's family knows their child best and their usual or habitual speech pattern and behavior; when they think their child is behaving or speaking 'differently' they should always be listened to. If NCSE is a real possibility, an EEG should be undertaken and will fortunately be able to definitively confirm or refute the possibility of NCSE. It is important to record an EEG to confirm that the first time a child with epilepsy presents with an abrupt, subtle or dramatic change in behavior or communication that they are in NCSE. This may preclude having to obtain a repeat EEG each and every time the child re-presents with similar features and should ensure that the child is promptly diagnosed and treated.

Continuous spike-wave in slow-sleep is a difficult form of NCSE to diagnose because its manifestations may be so subtle. Most of the children with this disorder have established epilepsy, and usually, but not invariably, a focal epilepsy that is often being treated with carbamazepine. Their symptoms consist of decreased daytime neuro-psychological function; they do not learn as well at school or they have an important unexplained behavioral deterioration. The EEG during sleep shows what amount to NCSE, hence its name, CSWSS, and the clinical correlate is termed electrical status epilepticus of slow-wave sleep (ESESS). An EEG recorded during wakefulness may not necessarily suggest this disorder. A sleeping EEG – and one that records the deeper stages of sleep (when slow-wave sleep occurs) – is essential to make the diagnosis. Although this may sometimes be achieved during an outpatient EEG after a period of home sleep-deprivation or, rarely, following the use of melatonin, it is frequently necessary to admit the child for an overnight recording. Limited evidence suggests that CSWSS usually resolves spontaneously by adolescence, but if unrecognized (and untreated) in childhood will result in children sustaining irreversible cognitive impairment. Unfortunately, even successful treatment with 'normalization' of the EEG with resolution of CSWSS does not prevent this impairment. The difficulty and, often, dilemma in treating CSWSS is how 'aggressive' treatment should be; a range of treatments are available (ethosuximide, clobazam, prednisolone, sodium valproate, sulthiame, the ketogenic diet and even surgery) and there must be a clear rational approach to its treatment.

Landau–Kleffner syndrome is also considered by some, but not all clinicians, to represent a form of NCSE. This syndrome shares some features with the regression seen in autism and consequently (and unfortunately) is often regarded in the same light. As in all epilepsies, a clear history is important. In LKS, a previously 'normal' child presents with either focal seizures or a sudden and often dramatic deterioration in both receptive and expressive communication and social interaction. Children with this latter presentation are often considered to be deaf and referred for an ear, nose and throat (ENT) opinion. A waking EEG may show features that might initially suggest a diagnosis of benign partial epilepsy with centro-temporal spikes (BECTS), although a suspicious feature is that there is frequently bi-synchronous as well as focal activity in a child with LKS. Subsequently, a sleeping EEG will demonstrate marked sharp or spike and slow-wave activity over both temporal lobes. Seizures are relatively easy to control, unlike the communication and behavioral components. Treatment is similar to that in CSWSS, with prednisolone, sodium valproate, ethosuximide or clobazam (or any combination of these drugs), but more importantly, intensive speech and language therapy and neuro-psychological support may improve, but rarely normalize, the child's cognitive functioning and social interaction. Some children may respond to a specific surgical procedure, termed subpial transaction (or 'Morrell's procedure,' named after the clinician who first described the technique).

The treatment of NCSE is important and must be timely and appropriate. Excluding hypsarrhythmia occurring in infancy (discussed in earlier chapters), the treatment of NCSE begins with the correct diagnosis and is generally identical to that when treating CSE. However, it is important to understand that, rarely, the use of a benzodiazepine may convert NCSE into either tonic or even convulsive status epilepticus.

Unfortunately, episodes of NCSE recur frequently in a number of the symptomatic and genetic epilepsy syndromes or epilepsies and may last hours, days or weeks; occasionally the episodes stop spontaneously. NSCE may also be resistant to the anticonvulsants used to treat CSE. In these situations, other treatments, including short courses of prednisolone, intravenous levetiracetam or sodium valproate, rapid oral-loading with topiramate or the ketogenic diet may prove beneficial. Of these therapeutic options, the ketogenic diet may be more likely to result in a sustained benefit that may last days, weeks or longer. As yet, no clinical trials have addressed this issue.

Finally, it is important never to lose sight of the child and focus exclusively on treating their recurrent episodes of non-convulsive status with multiple drugs because this may have an even more deleterious effect on the child's ability to function and interact with their environment than the NCSE itself.

Epilepsia partialis continua (EPC)

Although this very rare epileptic phenomenon is not usually regarded as a form of status epilepticus, arguably it should be. As the term implies, it describes a child who is completely conscious but who shows continuous partial motor seizures which are typically manifest by myoclonic or clonic seizures that affect any part of the body and face and vary in both intensity and rhythm. The manifestations may be remarkably localized: for example, involving only one or two fingers or the thumb. Epilepsia partialis continua may last hours, days or weeks, or even longer. The usual causes include herpes simplex encephalitis (and other, rarer viral encephalitides), Rasmussen's syndrome, progressive neuronal degeneration of childhood (Alpers' disease), a mitochondrial cytopathy (specifically caused by a mutation in the POLG1 gene) and occasionally following a hypoxic–ischemic brain insult. In adult patients, phenytoin and phenobarbital are reported to be effective on occasions but in the authors' experience, pediatric EPC is invariably resistant to treatment, and consequently it tends to be treated with almost all known anticonvulsant treatments, including high-dose steroids and intravenous immunoglobulins; the latter may result in some temporary response. There is very limited information on the efficacy of the newest anticonvulsants in EPC. Hemispherectomy is the current treatment of choice in treating Rasmussen's syndrome in children; resective neurosurgery may also be indicated where there is an obvious structural lesion. Children with EPC are often managed on intensive care units and may be treated with infusions of either thiopentone, high-dose midazolam or propofol; unfortunately, although EPC may resolve, it will typically recur as these medications are withdrawn. In addition, both thiopentone and propofol may be complicated by significant and potentially fatal side effects. This again emphasizes the point that the focus of treatment must be the child and not just the seizures, in this case EPC.

ADDITIONAL READING

Chin RF, Verlust L, Neville BGR, Peters MJ, Scott RC. Inappropriate emergency management of status epilepticus in children contributes to need for intensive care. *J Neurol Neurosurg Psychiatry* 2004; **75**: 1584–88.

Walker M, Cross H, Smith S, *et al.* Nonconvulsive status epilepticus: Epilepsy Research Foundation workshop reports. *Epileptic Disord* 2005; **7**: 253–96.

Riviello JJ, Ashwal S, Hirtz D, *et al.* Practice parameter: diagnostic assessment of the child with status epilepticus (an evidence-based review): report of the Quality Standards Subcommittee of the Child Neurology Society. *Neurology* 2006; **67**: 1542–50.

Chin RF, Neville BG, Scott RC. Incidence, cause and short-term outcome of convulsive status epilepticus in childhood: prospective population-based study. *Lancet* 2006; **368**: 222–9.

Hussain N, Appleton R, Thorburn K. Etiology, course and outcome of children admitted to pediatric intensive care with convulsive status epilepticus: a retrospective 5-year review. *Seizure* 2007; **16**: 305–12.

Raspall-Chaure M, Chin RF, Neville BG, Bedford H, Scott RC. The epidemiology of convulsive status epilepticus in children: a critical review. *Epilepsia* 2007; **48**: 1652–63.

Appleton R, Macleod S, Martland T. Drug management for acute tonic-clonic convulsions including convulsive status epilepticus in children. *Cochrane Database Syst Rev* 2008; **16**: CD001905 (Review).

Chin RFM, Neville BGR, Peckham C, *et al.* Treatment of community-onset, childhood convulsive status epilepticus: a prospective, population-based study. *Lancet Neurol* 2008; **7**: 696–703.

Lewena S, Pennington V, Acworth J, *et al.* Emergency management of pediatric convulsive status epilepticus: a multicenter study of 542 patients. *Pediatr Emerg Care* 2009; **25**: 83–7.

Singh RK, Gaillard WD. Status epilepticus in children. *Curr Neurol Neurosci Rep* 2009; **9**: 137–44.

7

The prevention of epilepsy and its consequences

Richard Appleton and Peter Camfield

The concept of the prevention of epilepsy has received relatively little attention, including within the area of epilepsy research. The majority of animal-based research has focused on both the induction and pathogenesis of chronic, drug resistant epilepsy and subsequent attempts to identify new treatments. The paucity of research in the prevention of epilepsy is particularly surprising in view of the largely accepted belief that at least 30% of 'epilepsy' in children is intractable and drug resistant. Furthermore, epilepsy in a significant proportion of this group will have arisen secondary to a post-natally acquired known cerebral insult, or a genetic disorder. In addition, the consequences of frequent and drug resistant seizures are significant, often resulting in physical, educational and behavioral complications.

Although it is inevitable that most seizures and epilepsies will not be preventable, which in a significant part reflects the major significant genetic influence in their pathogenesis, this does not and should not preclude attempts to try and reduce their incidence and their consequences.

The prevention of epilepsy can be considered on many levels, ranging from the initiation of the first seizure to the consequences of a wrong diagnosis of epilepsy or epilepsy syndrome, failure to identify an underlying cause and suboptimal management.

It would be both inappropriate and impossible to address all these potential areas of prevention in this chapter but some of the more important areas will be discussed as these are of relevance to those clinicians who regularly care for children with epilepsy and their families.

Prevention of a diagnosis of epilepsy

This section considers the following:
- prevention of a wrong diagnosis of seizures
- prevention of a wrong diagnosis of an epilepsy syndrome
- prevention of a wrong cause of epilepsy.

The management of children with epilepsy should always begin with correctly identifying the epileptic nature of the child's seizures, the accurate classification of the seizure type or types and epilepsy syndrome (wherever possible) and consideration and appropriate investigation of the epilepsy. From personal experience, it is surprising how many clinicians fail to consider why a child's epilepsy has occurred; in part this may reflect their belief that most epilepsy is 'idiopathic' – that it is 'one's own' (derived from the Greek word, '*idios*'), epilepsy which has somehow arisen in isolation and as a primary disease. While many epilepsies may be genuinely 'idiopathic' and almost certainly genetically determined, this is certainly not true for all the pediatric epilepsies. Failure to correctly identify the epileptic nature of the child's paroxysmal events, the correct epilepsy syndrome and a potentially treatable cause may have a significant and potentially irreversible effect on the child's care and future life. This necessitates that all clinicians who treat children with epilepsy must have an interest, ideally an enthusiasm, in treating epilepsy and be appropriately trained. They should also ensure that they remain up-to-date with advances in the diagnosis, genetics and specific treatments of the different epilepsy syndromes.

Prevention of the primary and severe (malignant) familial epilepsies

Primary and severe familial epilepsies include:
- progressive, neuro-degenerative epilepsies
- disease-specific epilepsy (e.g., tuberous sclerosis).

For obvious reasons it is important to identify specific genetically determined epilepsies, and particularly those that may be associated with a malignant or progressive course, because this will provide valuable and practical information for both prognostic advice and genetic counseling. Specific and important examples include the neuro-cutaneous syndromes (tuberous sclerosis and neuro-fibromatosis), Angelman and Rett syndromes, severe myoclonic epilepsy of infancy (Dravet syndrome), the lissencephaly syndromes, the neuronal ceroid lipofuscinoses and the mitochondrial cytopathies (e.g., progressive neuronal degeneration of childhood or Alpers' disease). Many of these disorders present within the first few years of life and hopefully will have been diagnosed before the birth of another sibling. Establishing an early diagnosis will at least provide the family with information that may help them decide on whether to embark on another pregnancy and an opportunity for elective pre-natal assessment, should this be available.

Prevention of the secondary causes of epilepsy

Secondary causes of epilepsy include:
- neonatal hypoxic–ischemic encephalopathy
- non-traumatic brain injury (meningitis/encephalitis)
- traumatic brain (head) injury
- febrile seizures and mesial temporal lobe epilepsy.

The neonatal period is the time of life with the highest risk of acute symptomatic seizures and the potential initiation of chronic epilepsy. In part this relates to the fact that the brain is relatively 'hyperexcitable' and therefore more likely to seize than in later childhood. The newborn brain is therefore more susceptible to a large number of cerebral and systemic insults, which may be transient or permanent. Neonatal hypoxic–ischemic cerebral injury, periventricular hemorrhage and hypoglycemia are particularly likely to give rise to an epilepsy that not only commences in early infancy (including West syndrome) but is also extremely difficult, if not impossible, to treat and is invariably associated with other, severe neurological impairments. To a certain extent, and specifically in developed countries, these conditions may be partly preventable by anticipating problems with high-risk pregnancies and by providing meticulous ante-, peri- and post-natal medical and nursing care.

Infections of the central nervous system (CNS) are common in children and particularly in infancy (including the neonatal period) and early childhood. Acute symptomatic seizures may be one of the presenting features of both meningitis and encephalitis and epilepsy may complicate both infections, with the risk of late epilepsy being 10% in meningitis and 20% in encephalitis. There is no doubt that the earlier the diagnosis and initiation of appropriate treatment the better the outcome and this relates to both survival and morbidity, including epilepsy. Epilepsy that arises as a sequel to meningitis and encephalitis typically includes focal and generalized seizures and is usually difficult to treat, and this again justifies all attempts to reduce its incidence. This will clearly include public health measures (and specifically improved immunization rates for all transmissible disease including measles, tuberculosis, HIV and malaria) and an improved diagnosis and treatment of meningitis and encephalitis.

Traumatic brain injury remains one of the most common causes of epilepsy, particularly in mid-childhood and adolescence. Most studies suggest that approximately 12–15% of children who have experienced a moderate or severe head injury will develop post-traumatic epilepsy (PTE), a figure approximately 15 times greater than the normal, non-head-injured pediatric population. Mild or minor head injuries are not associated with an increased risk of late epilepsy. Risk factors for late PTE are directly related to the severity of the head injury, duration of post-traumatic amnesia and the occurrence of early epileptic seizures in the first week after the head injury. Clearly, numerous attempts have been and continue to be made to reduce the incidence of head injuries. There have also been significant advances in acute resuscitation; however, increased survival is often at the expense of increased morbidity, including PTE. There is active research in the development and use of neuro-protective drugs and techniques that may reduce the impact of not only the primary (traumatic) brain injury but also the secondary effects of cerebral edema, hypoxic–ischemic changes and epileptogenesis. Despite several large, well-designed studies, there is no evidence that the use of prophylactic anticonvulsants taken immediately after the head injury (including before any early epileptic seizure) will prevent the development of late PTE. Considerably more work needs to be undertaken to reduce the incidence of PTE and this must include the prevention of head injuries. There is no doubt that the legal requirement to use seat belts and the increasingly credible and acceptable use of bicycle helmets has resulted in a significant reduction in head injuries and its consequences, including PTE. However, more can and should be done. In respect of road traffic accidents this could include increasing the age of obtaining a driving licence (currently 17 years in the UK). Other options, as in many parts of Canada and the USA, include an approach not to increase the age of driving but rather the concept of graduated licences, whereby young people are not allowed to drive without another licensed driver in the car for a number of months, driving is not permitted after midnight for a year and there is a limit on the number of passengers that can be in the car. Additional measures could include increased penalties for dangerous driving and improved and more widespread 'traffic-calming' or 'traffic-slowing' measures in towns and cities.

The entity of 'febrile seizures' remains an enigma and it is possible that the traditional understanding and teaching of febrile seizures may be radically reviewed with further advances in the pathogenesis of hyperthermia (fever)-induced seizures and in molecular genetics. Evidence for this has been inspired by the identification of the genetic epilepsy syndrome of generalized epilepsy and febrile seizures 'plus' (GEFS+). In addition, there is the ongoing controversy regarding the possible causative association of complex febrile seizures (those that last longer than 15 minutes, or those with clear unilateral or focal features) and the later development of temporal lobe epilepsy (TLE). Approximately 3% of all children with febrile seizures will have an afebrile seizure by seven years of age, and this figure rises to approximately 8% by 25 years of age. Conversely, it is estimated that between 30 and 70% of individuals with temporal lobe epilepsy will have a history of febrile seizures in infancy, and these will usually have been complex in nature, including febrile status epilepticus. Temporal lobe epilepsy is often resistant to anticonvulsant treatment and is frequently associated with additional cognitive and psychological impairments. Although surgery is frequently effective (if not curative of the epilepsy), not every individual with TLE will be a surgical candidate; in addition, there is still a limited availability worldwide of accredited centres for epilepsy surgery, particularly in children. Both animal and, more recently, human evidence suggest that the process of epileptogenesis (the induction of chronic epilepsy) may have an onset at, or very soon after, an episode of febrile status epilepticus. This clearly raises important issues about both the importance of the termination of a first episode of febrile status epilepticus as rapidly as possible and the use of rescue or emergency medication rapidly for out-of-hospital use to try and prevent a further episode. The successful treatment of a first or subsequent prolonged episode of febrile status may have important implications for the prevention of the late development of temporal lobe epilepsy caused by mesial temporal sclerosis. Although this is unlikely to lead to the routine use of anticonvulsant prophylaxis after a first febrile seizure, it may lead to a more aggressive treatment approach to terminate a febrile seizure, and specifically the early use of out-of-hospital rescue medication, including by paramedic ambulance staff. Recent data have suggested that this may be effective and this may be facilitated by a change in the preferred out-of-hospital rescue medication from rectal diazepam to buccal midazolam, which as well as being more effective, may be more acceptable to the child's carers (1). However, these hypotheses need to be confirmed by additional long-term data which will hopefully be subsequently reported from the initial 'FEBSTAT' study in the US (2).

Prevention of a wrong treatment of epilepsy

This section considers the following:
- status epilepticus
- seizure types/epilepsy syndromes
- chronic epilepsy
- the cognitive, behavioral and social consequences of chronic epilepsy.

The following aspects of prevention again emphasize the common underlying principle which is that all clinicians involved in the care of children with epilepsy should be interested and appropriately trained.

Although the outcome of convulsive status epilepticus (CSE) is often directly related to the underlying cause, its duration and management are also important. Consequently, the under- or over-treatment of CSE may have irreversible consequences, not only contributing to a temporary deterioration in seizure control but also, more importantly, to the induction of a state of chronic epilepsy. Guidelines exist for the management of CSE and although these differ between the US, Canada and the UK, it is important to be aware that they are largely evidence-based with their primary role being to terminate the episode rapidly and safely. The guidelines comprise clear recommendations about which drugs to give and in what doses, and importantly, with specific clear timings of when to give the drugs and when to move on to the next treatment step. As mentioned previously, the more aggressive treatment of seizures, both febrile and afebrile, including out-of-hospital treatment, may help to prevent the incidence of prolonged and refractory convulsive status and, possibly, the development of later temporal lobe epilepsy. Clearly, treatment must be appropriate and not over-aggressive to prevent any iatrogenic complications. These issues are discussed in more detail in the 'Status epilepticus' and 'Risks and hazards of epilepsy' chapters.

The prevention of the many potential cognitive, emotional and social consequences of chronic epilepsy is difficult and outside the scope of this chapter. Many of these consequences will depend on the specific epilepsy and underlying cause. However, it is important to understand that the appropriate and optimal management of these children will also have an impact on these outcomes, as will society's response to epilepsy as a neurological disorder. The management of chronic epilepsy is characteristically difficult and importantly the approach should not simply be one of increasing the doses of pre-existing anticonvulsants, or by adding another anticonvulsant. Children with chronic epilepsy are subject to many different types of seizure, often occurring on a daily or weekly basis, and they will invariably have additional difficulties, including in their education and social functioning. The risk of using multiple anticonvulsants or 'polypharmacy' is greatest in this population with the additional (and potentially greater) risk of causing significant adverse side effects, particularly on the CNS, which may result in sedation and attention and memory difficulties. Sedation is a potent trigger to reducing seizure-threshold which may further increase seizure frequency and a spiraling escalation of the child's difficulties. This emphasizes the importance of a holistic approach, treating the child and not just trying to achieve total seizure freedom, which is rarely possible in this specific population. Arguably, the primary objective, if not principle, should be one of substitution or replacement monotherapy, rather than polytherapy or 'polypharmacy.' While there is relatively good evidence that two anticonvulsant drugs may be more effective than a single drug (and without causing any unacceptable side effects), it is important to recognize that, apart from a few anecdotal exceptions, there are no published data (and therefore evidence) that three anticonvulsant drugs are generally more effective than two. Consequently, if seizure control is poor in a child who is already receiving two antiepileptic drugs, and a third is to be added, the aim should be one of substitution or replacement and not simply addition. Unfortunately this is often far easier said than done.

REFERENCES

1. McIntyre J, Robertson S, Norris E, *et al.* Safety and efficacy of buccal midazolam versus rectal diazepam for emergency treatment of seizures in children: a randomized controlled trial. *Lancet* 2005; **366**: 205–10.
2. Shinnar S, Hesdorffer DC, Nordli DR Jr, *et al.* Phenomenology of prolonged febrile seizures: result of the FEBSTAT study. *Neurology* 2008; **71**: 170–6.

8

Medico-legal aspects of epilepsy

Richard Appleton and Peter Camfield

Children with epilepsy and their families deserve to receive the best available service from their healthcare professionals to ensure accurate diagnoses and optimal care. The objective is to try and maximize their quality of life and minimize the consequences of the disorder and its treatment, and this should be the primary and over-riding aim of everyone who is responsible for the specialist care of all children with epilepsy, irrespective of whether the children are seen in a general pediatric, pediatric neurology or pediatric epilepsy clinic. Unfortunately, the consequences of poor and less than appropriate standards of care may have effects on more than the children themselves, or their families. Predictably, these may include legal consequences, a number of which regularly result in successful litigation for the plaintiff and against the medical institutions and clinicians. These issues include:

- **The incorrect diagnosis of epilepsy**. This cannot be over-emphasized, as will have been evident throughout this book. Epilepsy continues to be both under- but also over-diagnosed. A cardiac arrhythmia is the most important non-epileptic paroxysmal event that should not be missed, as this is treatable. Conversely, if not diagnosed the next episode of cardiac syncope may result in death, or severe and irreversible brain injury. Simple syncope (faints), self-gratification (masturbation), psychogenic non-epileptic seizures, parasomnias (including night terrors and sleep-walking), motor tics and rage attacks (also known as 'episodic dyscontrol syndrome') are the most common paroxysmal events that are frequently misdiagnosed as epileptic seizures. Infantile spasms and focal seizures arising from the frontal but also the temporal lobe (particularly in children under five or six years of age) are the most commonly missed seizure (epilepsy) diagnoses. Both a missed diagnosis of epilepsy as well as a wrong diagnosis of epilepsy may have significant and long-lasting effects on a person's life and, understandably, the individual and their family may feel aggrieved and angry and seek recompense.

Childhood Epilepsy: Management from Diagnosis to Remission, ed. Richard Appleton and Peter Camfield. Published by Cambridge University Press. © Cambridge University Press 2011.

- **The inaccurate classification of the child's epileptic seizures**. Common confusion arises between myoclonic seizures and infantile spasms and also between juvenile absences and focal (complex partial) seizures. Absence seizures that occur in juvenile absence and juvenile myoclonic epilepsy are usually less frequent, and typically last longer than in childhood-onset absence epilepsy. In addition, during the seizures, children and teenagers may continue talking (although it may be non-fluent or incoherent at times) and demonstrate semi-purposeful behavior, features that may lead to an incorrect diagnosis of a partial (focal) seizure. There are clinical implications of such inaccuracies; first, the child may be prescribed the wrong anticonvulsant, specifically carbamazepine or phenytoin, which may exacerbate the seizures; and second (as a consequence), the child's seizures will be potentially labeled as being intractable, leading to the prescription of additional (and unnecessary) anticonvulsants with obvious consequences. The young person and their family may also be given inappropriate – and incorrect – advice about their future career and employment opportunities if their epilepsy is labeled as being 'intractable.'
- **The failure to recognize non-convulsive (electrical) status epilepticus (NCSE)**. Non-convulsive status epilepticus is not the medical emergency that convulsive status is, but it may still have detrimental effects. Although the majority of these effects are not life-threatening they will, at the very least, affect concentration and memory (with significant educational implications). NCSE may also predispose children to feeding difficulties and aspiration, which could have major respiratory consequences.
- **The over-interpretation of the key investigations in epilepsy**. The EEG and the computed tomography (CT) and magnetic resonance imaging (MRI) brain scan are the most commonly undertaken investigations in epilepsy and their interpretation is likely to have a significant impact on making clinical decisions. It remains a commonly held belief that the EEG is a 'black and white' investigation, in that if the EEG is normal the child's paroxysmal episodes cannot represent an epileptic seizure and, conversely, if abnormal the episodes must be epileptic in origin. Those responsible for the interpretation of a child's EEG and its electro-clinical report must be adequately trained and understand the normal appearances of EEGs from the neonatal period and throughout childhood, as well as having the knowledge and experience of the EEG in the many pediatric epilepsy syndromes. Similar principles apply to neuro-imaging and particularly brain MRI with the need to correctly identify normal variants but also abnormalities, including developmental and acquired lesions. This is particularly the case with low-resolution (0.5 Tesla) MRI scanners.
- **The failure to consider and appropriately look for an underlying cause for the epilepsy**. This is particularly important where the cause is treatable or has genetic (counseling) implications, or both. Specific examples include hypoglycemia/hypocalcemia in neonates and infants, pyridoxine-dependency, tuberous sclerosis or neurofibromatosis type 1, a genetic syndrome (ring chromosome 20, Rett or Angelman syndrome), a cerebral tumor and the neuronal ceroid lipofuscinoses. It is of both interest and concern that a number of clinicians do

not appreciate that the diagnostic process in epilepsy is not complete until a cause for the epilepsy has at least been considered, investigated and, where appropriate, excluded.

- **The prescription of inappropriate antiepileptic medication.** This is clearly important because it may result in the child or young person experiencing continuing and unnecessary seizures with all the implications of uncontrolled seizures (physical injury, psychological stress, social isolation and stigmatization). This risk can be significantly reduced by correctly identifying and classifying the seizure type(s) and epilepsy syndrome. Vigabatrin is one of the anticonvulsants of choice for treating infantile spasms but it commonly exacerbates myoclonic (and absence) seizures. Carbamazepine, arguably the anticonvulsant of 'choice' in treating focal (partial) seizures, typically exacerbates absences (and myoclonic) seizures and may precipitate absence or myoclonic status; the same is true of phenytoin, which is relatively commonly prescribed to treat focal seizures in the USA.

- **The inappropriate management of convulsive status epilepticus (CSE).** The consequences of the inappropriate (over- or under-) management of CSE may be extremely serious, resulting in death or irreversible brain damage. Currently, this is one of the more common issues frequently leading to successful litigation. Clear national status guidelines exist within the UK, as endorsed by the Advanced Pediatric Life Support (APLS) programme and the Royal College of Pediatrics and Child Health (RCPCH) (1). Close adherence to these guidelines should minimize, if not obviate, successful litigation.

- **Failure to give appropriate and accurate information to families.** The range of topics and the extent of information are clearly extensive. These include: the potential risks from seizures (including in causing physical injury and even, in certain circumstances, death); the side effects of any antiepileptic medication that is prescribed (including Stevens–Johnson syndrome or severe skin exfoliation with carbamazepine and lamotrigine, probable irreversible visual field constriction with vigabatrin and the teratogenic effects of a number of drugs); the potential complications of known drug interactions (specifically the interaction of many antiepileptic drugs with the oral contraceptive [potentially, with very serious consequences]); career and driving licence information. The topic of sudden unexpected death in epilepsy (SUDEP), and when and how this should be discussed with the family, remains controversial, although probably more within the adult rather than pediatric forum. Guidelines have been published on how to most appropriately discuss SUDEP (2, 3) for parents of children with epilepsy.

This above list is clearly not comprehensive. It is also not intended to be and should not be perceived as an *aide mémoire* or 'check list' to practise defensive medicine. However, these important issues should be perceived and interpreted as providing a framework for establishing and developing the type of epilepsy service that should be the gold standard and the one that should underpin all epilepsy clinics operating within secondary and tertiary care units. It also highlights the importance of close liaison with tertiary pediatric epilepsy units to obtain early advice for those children in whom the diagnosis of recurrent paroxysmal events is unclear and those who fail to respond to the first two antiepileptic drugs. Finally, it should also be regarded as a justification for the development of closer links and the establishment of 'networks' within and between secondary and tertiary care units. This practice and network principle is similar to the recommendations outlined in the guideline documents published by both the National Institute for Health and Clinical Excellence (NICE) (4) in England and Wales and the Scottish Intercollegiate Guidelines Network (SIGN) in Scotland (5). The benefits of such networks include not only clinical improvements (discussing difficult patients) but also educational improvement (disseminating and sharing information on new antiepileptic drugs, genetic advances and specific management guidelines) and providing opportunities for audit and research (6).

REFERENCES

1. *Advanced Pediatric Life Support: The Practical Approach* 2nd edn. London and Oxford, BMJ Books and Blackwells Publishing 2005.
2. Appleton RE. Mortality in pediatric epilepsy. *Arch Dis Childhood* 2003; **88**: 1091–4.
3. Gayatri NA, Morrall MCHJ, Jain V, *et al.* Parental and physician beliefs regarding the provision and content of written sudden unexpected death in epilepsy (SUDEP) information. *Epilepsia* 2010; **51**: 777–82.
4. National Institute for Health and Clinical Excellence (NICE). The epilepsies: the diagnosis and management of the epilepsies in adults and children in primary and secondary care. Clinical Guideline 20. *NICE* October 2004; www.nice.org.uk.
5. Scottish Intercollegiate Guidelines Network (SIGN). Diagnosis and management of epilepsies in children and young people. Guideline 81. *SIGN* March 2005; www.sign.ac.uk.
6. Appleton RE, The Mersey Region Pediatric Epilepsy Interest Group. Seizure-related injuries in children with newly diagnosed and untreated epilepsy. *Epilepsia* 2002; **43**: 764–7.

Glossary

Seizure

An epileptic seizure is an intermittent, stereotyped disturbance of function, manifest as altered consciousness, behavior, emotion, motor function, sensation or perception which may occur in isolation or in any combination and that on clinical grounds results from abnormal or excessive cortical neuronal discharges. Epilepsy is not a single disease entity but a symptom of an underlying neurological disorder.

Seizure characteristics

Aura – subjective experience that precedes a complex partial or secondarily generalized seizure, usually only for a few seconds. An aura is a simple partial seizure and the symptoms depend on which brain area the seizure begins. Most arise from the temporal, occipital or parietal lobes; auras are uncommon in frontal lobe seizures.

Automatism – movements that occur during a complex partial or absence seizure that are semi-purposeful but without useful function at that time. Some automatisms may be quite sophisticated and prolonged and can occur both in the absence seizures seen in juvenile absence epilepsy and in the complex partial seizures of temporal lobe epilepsy.

Provoked seizure – a seizure that is the result of an acute, transient brain disturbance.

Psychogenic, non-epileptic seizure (PNES; also called a pseudo-epileptic seizure, or less usefully, a pseudo-seizure) – a seizure that has no recognizable abnormal simultaneous electrical discharge in the brain and is psychogenic in origin. Most PNES resemble a prolonged tonic-clonic seizure and it is generally easy to differentiate a psychogenic, non-epileptic seizure from a genuine, tonic-clonic epileptic seizure without the need for confirmatory video–EEG evidence on the basis of a good history and out-of-hospital video recordings.

Todd's paresis – weakness following a seizure that lasts less than 24 hours and manifests as a hemiparesis or as weakness of a single limb.

Triggered or reflex seizure – a seizure that occurs in response to a specific stimulus, a stimulus that would not be expected to trigger a seizure in normal people.

Unprovoked seizure – a seizure that occurs when brain function appears to be normal for the individual and there is no apparent provoking factor.

Seizure types

Generalized seizures

These are seizures that appear to begin suddenly and involve the whole brain, simultaneously. There is no warning or aura, loss of consciousness is immediate and if there are body movements they are typically bilateral and symmetrical. The ictal EEG suggests seizure onset throughout the brain, all at once. The clear division between generalized and focal (partial) seizures remains under debate.

Absence – a seizure characterized by sudden loss of consciousness, retention of posture, staring, minimal automatisms and sudden return of consciousness usually after ten to 20 seconds. There is no post-ictal confusion.

Astatic – similar to atonic ('akinetic' is not synonymous with astatic or atonic because 'akinetic' simply means no movement – and this can occur in an absence seizure).

Atonic – a seizure with sudden loss of consciousness and sudden loss of postural tone, as if a puppet's strings have been cut.

Clonic – repeated and rhythmic jerks that affect one or more limbs or the whole body and that usually last between 30 seconds and two minutes. These typically follow the tonic phase of a tonic-clonic seizure but may occur in isolation.

Myoclonus – seizures characterized by a single, sudden jerk of a muscle or group of muscles. It is most often bilateral but may involve a single limb – or the head and neck.

Tonic – a seizure characterized by sudden loss of consciousness and generalized tonic contraction, typically resulting in a child falling stiffly, as if a tree has been felled.

Tonic-clonic – a seizure (or convulsion) with no warning or aura, characterized by loss of consciousness followed by generalized stiffening and roughly symmetrical clonic movements of most voluntary muscles that usually last two to three minutes. Confusion, headache and a period of sleep commonly follow.

Focal or partial seizures (previously called localization-related seizures)

These are seizures that begin in one place in the brain with or without propagation to adjacent areas or throughout the entire brain.

Complex partial – a seizure that starts in a localized brain area and spreads to involve sufficient brain area that consciousness is clouded or lost but does not continue to a generalized tonic-clonic seizure. Seizure duration is typically < 90

seconds although post-ictal confusion may last much longer. Most, but not all, complex partial seizures begin in the temporal lobe.

Partial (focal) with secondary generalization – a seizure that starts in a localized area of the brain and spreads to involve most of the brain with generalized tonic and clonic manifestations. If the patient is awake and the seizure spreads slowly there will be an aura or warning. The aura is a simple partial seizure that evolves to secondary generalization. It is important to appreciate that, if the spread of the seizure is very rapid, the seizure may on first consideration appear to be a generalized tonic-clonic seizure.

Simple partial – a seizure that remains localized to one area of the brain with preserved consciousness.

Epileptic spasms

A seizure characterised by a sudden generalised increase in muscle tone associated with extension, or flexion, of the arms and drop of the head. The spasms typically occur in a cluster with either a few or up to many dozens in a cluster. When they occur in infancy ($<$13 months of age), they are called infantile spasms. Spasms tend to be classified as a generalized seizure type, although there is clear evidence that in many patients (including those with tuberous sclerosis and unilateral structural lesions) the seizures originate in one area of the brain and rapidly spread across the corpus callosum, giving the appearance of a generalized spasm.

Epilepsy syndrome

A specific disorder characterized by the age at onset of seizures, the seizure type (or types), a characteristic EEG appearance (ictal and inter-ictal), a proposed etiology and a relatively well-defined prognosis and clinical course.

Specific syndrome characteristics

Febrile seizure (febrile convulsion) – a specific disorder with seizures occurring between six (and certainly 12) months and five years of age in a child with fever but without evidence of an infection of the central nervous system (CNS). There has been reluctance to define febrile seizures as an epilepsy syndrome because all seizures are provoked by a fever and the outcome is generally (but not universally) benign. Simple febrile seizures are defined as generalized tonic-clonic, brief ($<$ 15 minutes) and only occur once during a 24-hour period; complex febrile seizures are defined as either focal, prolonged ($>$ 15 minutes) or recurrent within a 24-hour period. Simple febrile seizures are followed by epilepsy in 2–3%, while the risk after complex febrile seizures is greater, in the range of five to 15%.

Focal, partial or localization-related epilepsies – epilepsy syndromes characterized by focal seizures. Focal syndromes may be idiopathic, symptomatic or crypto-genic (presumed symptomatic).

Generalized epilepsies – epilepsy syndromes characterized by generalized seizures only. Generalized epilepsy syndromes may be idiopathic, symptomatic or crypto-genic (presumed symptomatic).

Groups of epilepsy syndromes

Benign epilepsies – epilepsy syndromes characterized by relatively easy seizure control, spontaneous remission and good developmental outcome without neurological sequelae. While the prognosis is typically excellent, some patients with 'benign' epilepsies have unsatisfactory cognitive or social outcome.

Catastrophic or malignant epilepsies – epilepsies that result in developmental regression or stagnation. The term may be used interchangeably with 'epileptic encephalopathy.' The term may also be used to describe additional epilepsies characterized by very frequent seizures, including migrating partial seizures (epilepsy) in infancy and Rasmussen syndrome.

Cryptogenic epilepsy – an epilepsy without a known cause and no suspicion of a genetic cause. The term 'cryptogenic' (as in 'cryptic crossword'), originates from the Greek word 'Kryptos,' which means 'hidden' or 'origin unknown.' The use of this term may not be helpful because it is very dependent on the sophistication of investigations, especially brain imaging. An alternative term, 'presumed symptomatic,' is clumsy although it encourages clinicians to continue efforts to identify the underlying cause.

Idiopathic epilepsy – an epilepsy with no apparent structural brain problem, no associated intellectual or neurological deficit and a definite or presumed genetic cause.

Mesial temporal sclerosis (MTS) – refers to gliosis (scarring) and neuronal loss in mesial temporal lobe structures, particularly the hippocampus. This is often proposed to be caused by a very prolonged febrile seizure or repeated briefer seizures, especially if there is a pre-existing abnormality in the affected temporal lobe. Mesial temporal sceloris is typically associated with intractable epilepsy with associated cognitive and behavioral sequelae although the 'intractability' may not become apparent until around eight to ten years of age. Surgical resection in childhood is usually indicated and successful, and may prevent some cognitive and behavioral sequelae.

Symptomatic epilepsy – an epilepsy caused by an identified structural, genetic or biochemical abnormality.

Status epilepticus

Status epilepticus (convulsive) – a continuous seizure lasting for > 30 minutes characterized by generalized or localized clonic movements, usually with loss of awareness. It is important to emphasize that most convulsive seizures that last more than five minutes will, without pharmacological intervention, continue and meet the definition of convulsive status epilepticus. Also included within this definition are shorter, serial or cluster seizures which recur with no return of consciousness (between each seizure) for at least 30 minutes.

Status epilepticus – epilepsia partialis continua (EPC) – a focal seizure lasting at least 60 minutes (by some definitions), but usually far longer, up to many hours or even days or months, characterized by focal clonic movements affecting the face, a limb or collection of limbs, with retained consciousness.

Status epilepticus (non-convulsive, also sometimes termed 'electrical') – a continuous seizure lasting for > 30 minutes without convulsive manifestations and consciousness that may be impaired or lost. The most common types include absence, myoclonic or partial (focal), hypsarrhythmia and continuous spike-wave of slow-sleep (CSWSS).

Diagnosis

Channelopathy – a disorder of a membrane ion channel (usually inherited as an autosomal dominant trait and rarely as an autosomal recessive trait, or as a sporadic event). Sodium, potassium and calcium channels may be involved, depending on the specific epilepsy. Some channelopathies result in the same epilepsy disorder among affected individuals (for example, benign familial neonatal convulsions), while others may produce varying epilepsy syndromes, even within the same family (typically seen in generalized epilepsy with febrile seizures plus [GEFS+] and some of the idiopathic generalized epilepsies). Predictably, there is an overlap with other paroxysmal, but non-epileptic, movement disorders.

Epilepsy – a brain disorder characterized by recurrent unprovoked seizures. Epilepsy cannot be diagnosed after a first unprovoked seizure because only 50% will have a recurrence. It is usually diagnosed after two unprovoked seizures, because following two, a recurrence can be expected in 80–90% of children.

Epileptic encephalopathy – an epilepsy characterized by frequent clinically apparent seizures or a markedly abnormal EEG (typically spike and wave, polyspike and wave or hypsarrhythmia) without any obvious clinically apparent seizures and associated with decreased cognitive function that is often irreversible. The more 'common' examples include Ohtahara syndrome, West syndrome, severe myoclonic epilepsy of infancy (Dravet syndrome), Landau–Kleffner syndrome, continuous spike-wave of slow-sleep (CSWSS) and Lennox–Gastaut syndrome.

Video–EEG telemetry – this is the simultaneous video recording of a child's clinical seizures or paroxysmal events (whatever their nature) and their EEG. It is an in-patient investigation and may be recorded using surface (scalp) or, far less frequently, intracranial electrodes. Its main role is in the pre-surgical evaluation of children with suspected focal epilepsy. It is also invaluable in the investigation of children with difficult-to-diagnose waking, or nocturnal paroxysmal events or possible psychogenic, non-epileptic seizures. For some patients it permits a more accurate epilepsy syndrome diagnosis and may contribute to an understanding of how many, very subtle or unwitnessed seizures a child is having. It is generally not a substitute or replacement for a good clinical history and for many patients an inexpensive home video may be equally helpful.

Electroencephalography (EEG)

EEG background – the EEG rhythms that are recorded when a person is awake and relaxed or asleep but not having a seizure.

Photosensitivity – an abnormal spike or polyspike (usually with a slow-wave) discharge provoked by intermittent photic stimulation during an EEG recording. All routine EEG recordings should use this provocation technique. The usual flash frequency inducing a photosensitive (photoparoyxsmal) response is 18–30 Hz. Not all people with photosensitivity on EEG have epilepsy. It is most commonly seen in the idiopathic generalized epilepsies, and specifically juvenile myoclonic epilepsy. Rarely, 'normal' individuals may demonstrate a pure photosensitive epilepsy, one of the reflex epilepsies. As an electro-clinical phenomenon, it is most commonly seen in individuals between 12 and 20 years of age and particularly in females. A very rare photosensitive-like phenomenon may be seen in children with late infantile neuronal ceroid lipofuscinosis ('Batten's disease') when the child demonstrates a whole-body myoclonic seizure in response to a flash frequency of just 1 Hz and not at faster flash frequencies.

Polyspike discharge – multiple (usually two) spikes that may or may not be followed by a slow wave and which are often associated with myoclonic seizures.

Spike discharge – a sharp wave that lasts less than 80 milliseconds that may be localized or generalized and is considered to reflect an increased risk of epilepsy. A rhythmic 'spike and wave' discharge is considered to be the electrical hallmark of epilepsy.

Treatment

Antiepileptic drug (AED; also called an anticonvulsant) – a drug used for the treatment of epilepsy. In part the term is inappropriate because none of the current AEDs prevents epilepsy – they simply suppress seizures but do not seem to affect the prognosis or natural history of the epilepsy.

Ketogenic diet – a comprehensive but unnatural diet used for the treatment of epilepsy. Most of the diet's calories are derived from fat, the protein content is limited to that necessary for growth and minimal carbohydrates are allowed. There are broadly three variants: the classical (largely food-based); the medium chain triglyceride (MCT – mainly liquid-based); and the modified Atkins diet (the least restricting for both child and family). Approximately one-third of children with intractable epilepsy will respond for a substantial period of time, although a significant number will subsequently relapse.

Vagus (or vagal) nerve stimulator (VNS) – this is an implanted device the size of an average wrist watch that electrically stimulates the left vagus nerve in the neck. It has been shown to reduce seizure frequency in approximately one-third of patients, irrespective of seizure type. Complete seizure freedom is unusual and it is usually used for children whose epilepsy is refractory to antiepileptic drugs but who are not candidates for cortical resection epilepsy surgery.

Clinical course

Intractable or medically refractory epilepsy – a definition that continues to be debated. Operationally, it is an epilepsy that fails to respond to appropriate medication – usually defined as failure to respond to maximally tolerated doses of two (at most, three) AEDs – as well as never achieving a seizure-free period of 12 months. During long follow-up studies occasional patients are identified who have several years of complete remission from seizures followed by uncontrollable epilepsy, therefore the definitional requirement of 'never achieving a seizure-free period of 12 months' is questionable.

Remission – epilepsy is usually said to be in remission if there have been no seizures for either two to five years with or without ongoing treatment with an antiepileptic drug. Many epidemiological studies distinguish between remission with or without ongoing medication treatment. For most patients and families, the concept is most poignant if the remission is without medication. The term 'spontaneous remission' can only be used in those children who remain seizure-free after the antiepileptic dug has been discontinued or who were never treated but became seizure-free.

Sudden unexplained (or unexpected) death in epilepsy (SUDEP) – this term describes the circumstance when a person with epilepsy dies without an identifiable cause noted clinically or at autopsy (post-mortem). The definition is confusing because the terms 'sudden' and 'unexpected' are almost synonymous. For this reason, possibly 'unexplained' is preferred to 'unexpected.' In children SUDEP is extremely rare. The mechanisms of SUDEP remain unknown and may be multiple, although respiratory suppression or a cardiac arrhythmia induced by a seizure are the most likely causes.

Index

absence epilepsy *see* childhood absence epilepsy;
    juvenile absence epilepsy
absence status 128–9
absences (absence seizures) 32–3, 39–40
    atypical, Dravet syndrome 12
    differential diagnosis 40
accidental deaths 47, 109–10
accidents 47–8, 109–10
acetazolamide 96
ACTH therapy 17–18, 62–3
acute presentation of seizures 30–1
acute symptomatic seizures 1, 5, 30
adherence *see* compliance
adolescent-onset epilepsies 73–105
    cognitive and social outcomes 99–100
    common epilepsy syndromes 79–88
    diagnostic problems 74–9
    drug treatment 88–92
    restrictions 92
    treatment 95–9
    triggers 92–5
adolescents
    effects of puberty on established epilepsy 74
    incidence of epilepsy 73–4, 74
    management of cognitive and behavior
        problems 101
    transition to adult epilepsy services 102–4
adrenoleucodystrophy 88
adverse effects of antiepileptic drugs *see* side effects
    of antiepileptic drugs
adversive seizures 37
alcohol use 93–4
Alpers' disease 16, 22, 116
anger, paroxysmal 36–7
anoxic epileptic seizure 34

anoxic seizures, reflex 2, 34, 76
antidepressants, interactions with 118
antiepileptic drugs (AEDs)
    adolescent-onset epilepsies 88–92
    appropriate use 138, 141
    childhood-onset epilepsies 53–4, 54–5, 55
    combination therapy 22–3, 46, 89, 97, 138
    compliance or adherence 20, 45–6, 91–2
    duration of treatment 56–7, 90
    failure of first choice 22–3, 53
    further trials 58
    generic and proprietary forms 89–90
    infant-friendly formulations 16
    infantile epilepsies 15–16
    missed doses 46
    refractory epilepsy *see* intractable epilepsy
    relapse risk after withdrawal 57, 90, 112–13
    risks and hazards 115–19
    serum concentration monitoring 16, 46
    side-effects *see* side effects of antiepileptic drugs
    withdrawal 57, 90–1, 112–13
anxiety 49, 51, 120
astatic seizures 42
Atkins diet, modified 24
atonic seizures 42, 43
attention deficit hyperactivity disorder (ADHD)
    49, 50, 120
atypical benign partial epilepsy of
    childhood 58
aura 83–4, 85
autism 51–2
automatisms 84, 85
autonomic symptoms 41, 84
autosomal dominant nocturnal frontal lobe
    epilepsy (ADNFLE) 36

bathing 47, 109
Batten's disease 22
behavior problems 49, 50, 100, 121
    antiepileptic drug-related 118–19
    management in adolescents 101
behaviors, abnormal paroxysmal 36–8
benign epilepsy of childhood with centro-
        temporal spikes (BECTS) 3, 40–1
    management 55, 56
    onset of puberty and 74
    prognosis 63–4, 65, 66, 111
benign familial neonatal–infantile seizures 15
benign focal epilepsies of childhood 40–2
benign infantile epilepsies 14–15, 20, 26–7
benign infantile seizures 14–15, 26–7
benign myoclonic epilepsy of infancy 15, 27, 111
benign partial epilepsy with occipital paroxysms
        (BEOP) 41–2
benign rolandic epilepsy of childhood (BREC)
        see benign epilepsy of childhood with
        centro-temporal spikes
benzodiazepines
    infantile epilepsies 19
    prolonged seizures 115, 126
    side effects 118
    status epilepticus 113–14, 126, 130–1
bicycles 48, 109
biotinidase deficiency 9
blank spells 32–3
bone health 47–8, 94, 117
brain lesions, structural 6, 7–8
brain tumors 7, 24
burns 47–8, 109

calcium supplements 47–8, 94, 117
carbamazepine
    adolescent-onset epilepsies 81, 89, 95–6
    childhood-onset epilepsies 55
    exacerbation of seizures 52
    infantile epilepsies 16
    side effects 116
cardiac arrhythmias 77, 139
cardiogenic syncope 34, 77, 139
carpet burns 2
catamenial epilepsy 94
cataplexy 37
catastrophic epilepsy 6
cause of epilepsy, failure to look for underlying
        134, 140–1
channelopathies 12–13, 15
Charlie Foundation 62
child abuse 78
childhood absence epilepsy (CAE) 39–40

prognosis 64–5, 66, 80
childhood occipital epilepsy
    early-onset see Panayiotopoulos syndrome
    late-onset 41–2
childhood-onset epilepsies (2 to 12 years) 29–45
    acute presentation of seizures 30–1
    clinical history 29–30
    co-morbidities 48–52
    first-line medication 53, 54, 55
    later management 63
    middle management 45–55
    presentations and differential diagnoses 32
    prognosis 63–6
    relapse after withdrawal of medication 57
    safety restrictions 47–8
    specific epilepsies 39–44
chromosomal disorders 8
clinical presentation of epilepsy 1
clobazam
    adolescent-onset epilepsies 81, 89
    childhood-onset epilepsies 54, 55
    in Dravet syndrome 19
co-morbidities 21, 48–52, 99
cognitive delay 49–50
    see also developmental regression
cognitive effects of antiepileptic drugs 118–19
cognitive outcome, long-term 65–6, 99–100
compliance (adherence) 20, 45–6, 91–2
computed tomography (CT) 3–4, 31
congenital malformations 54, 117–18
coning 30
continuous spike-wave of slow-sleep (CSWSS) 38,
        52, 58, 129, 130
contraception 94–5
corpus callosotomy 60–1
cortical dysplasia 59
corticosteroid therapy 17–18, 62–3
cycling 48, 109

dentatorubro-pallidoluysian atrophy
        (DRPLA) 88
depression 49, 51, 78, 120
developmental regression
    in childhood epilepsies 38–9
    in Dravet syndrome 12, 26
    in infantile epilepsies 21
    in migrating partial seizures in infancy
        13–14
    in West syndrome 10–11, 21, 26
    see also learning difficulties
diagnosis of epilepsy 1–4
    childhood-onset epilepsies 29–30
    in adolescents 74–9

diagnosis of epilepsy (*cont.*)
  incorrect 139
  prevention of wrong 134
  reviewing 52
diazepam, rectal 115, 126
Doose syndrome *see* myoclonic–astatic epilepsy
Down syndrome (trisomy 21) 8, 21
Dravet syndrome (severe myoclonic
    epilepsy of infancy) 12–13
  ketogenic diet 25, 61
  prognosis 26, 111
  treatment 19, 20, 22, 58
drop attacks, epileptic 33, 42, 43, 109
drowning 47, 109
dual pathology 59
dysembryoblastic neuroepithelial tumor (DNET) 59

EEG *see* electroencephalography
electrical status epilepticus of slow-wave sleep
    (ESESS) 38, 130
  management 52, 62–3
  prognosis 66
electrocardiogram (ECG) 77
electroencephalography (EEG)
  invasive monitoring 59
  misinterpretation 52, 140
  role 2–3
encephalitis 135
epilepsia partialis continua (EPC) 131
epilepsy, defined 1
epilepsy surgery 23–4, 97–9, 61
  epilepsia partialis continua 131
  palliative 23, 60–1
  resective 23, 60
  withdrawal of medication after 57
epilepsy syndromes 3
  common, in early infancy 9–14
  presenting in adolescence 79–88
  presenting in childhood 39–44
  usefulness of concept 39
epilepsy with grand mal on awakening 79
epileptic encephalopathy 6, 42–4, 62–3
epileptic spasms 45
episodic dyscontrol disorder 36–7
ethosuximide 54
eyelid myoclonia with absences 40

falls 33
  non-epileptic 33
  with abnormal movements or convulsions 33–4
family
  adjustment 21, 121
  information provision 141

non-epileptic attack disorder 77–8
  transition to adult epilepsy services and
    103–4
family history 6
fear, paroxysmal 37
febrile seizures 5, 30–1
  Dravet syndrome 12
  investigations 30–1
  prevention 136–7
felbamate 54, 117
first aid, seizure 114
first unprovoked seizures 2, 110–11
focal (partial) epilepsies
  adolescent-onset 82–6, 95–6
  childhood-onset 58
  social and cognitive outcomes 100–1
  see also idiopathic partial epilepsies;
    symptomatic partial epilepsies
focal (partial) seizures
  absences 40
  in adolescents 83
  in childhood 33, 37
  in infants 5
  with normal imaging 44
folic acid supplements 54, 94, 118
fosphenytoin 127
fractures 47–8
frontal lobe epilepsy/seizures 36, 85–6
functional neuro-imaging 85

GABA-B gene mutations 13
gabapentin
  focal epilepsies 55, 95–6
  side effects 118
  worsening of epilepsy 53
GABRG2 gene mutations 42
generalized epilepsy with febrile seizures plus
    (GEFS+) 40, 42, 136
generalized tonic-clonic seizures (GTCS)
  in childhood absence epilepsy 40
  in infants 5
  in juvenile myoclonic epilepsy 79, 80
  versus syncope 34–5
genetic disorders 6
gingival hyperplasia 117
glucose transporter-1 (GLUT-1) deficiency 9, 14,
    24, 61

hallucinations 37
hazards of epilepsy *see* risks and hazards of
    epilepsy
head injuries 47–8, 109, 135–6
helmets 47, 109

hematological disorders, drug-induced 116
hemiconvulsion, hemiplegia and epilepsy (HHE) 113
history, clinical 2, 3, 29–30, 74–5
hormonal treatment, West syndrome 17–18, 23
hypoxic–ischemic encephalopathy, neonatal 20, 135
hypsarrhythmia 11, 129
    treatment 16, 17

idiopathic childhood occipital epilepsy of Gastaut 41–2
idiopathic generalized epilepsies (IGE)
    adolescent-onset 79–82
    childhood-onset 53–4, 65
    otherwise unclassifiable 79
idiopathic partial epilepsies, childhood-onset 53, 55, 64, 66
immunizations 20–1
inborn errors of metabolism 8–9, 22
incontinence 2
independence, limitations to 48
infantile epilepsies 5–27
    benign 14–15, 20, 26–7
    co-morbidities 21
    common syndromes 9–14
    early treatment 15–20
    epilepsy surgery 23–4
    family adjustment 21
    incidence 5
    ketogenic diet 24–5
    middle treatment 20–5
    prognosis 25–7
    symptomatic 6–9
infantile seizures, benign 14–15, 26–7
infantile spasms 5, 10, 11–12
    see also West syndrome
infections, central nervous system 135
information provision, to families 141
injuries, physical 47–8, 109–10
intellectual disability see learning difficulties
intensive care (therapy) unit 128, 131
intermittent explosive disorder 36–7
intracranial pressure, acutely raised 30
intractable (medically refractory) epilepsy 23, 57–8
    incorrect labeling 140
    perceived impact of 121–2
    predictors 64
    risk of 113
    see also epilepsy surgery
intravenous immunoglobulin (IVIG) 63, 131

juvenile absence epilepsy (JAE) 40, 79
    effect of puberty on incidence 73–4

prognosis 65
juvenile myoclonic epilepsy (JME) 79–82
    effect of puberty on incidence 73–4
    management 81–2
    outcomes 99–100, 111–12
    photosensitivity 87, 92
    risk of relapse 81–2, 112
    seizure types 40, 79
    versus progressive myoclonic epilepsy 86–7

ketogenic diet 24–5, 55, 61–2
    in adolescence 96
    in non-convulsive status epilepticus 131

lacosamide 55
Lafora body disease 87
lamotrigine
    adolescent-onset epilepsies 81, 89, 95–6
    childhood-onset epilepsies 53, 54, 55
    side effects 116
Landau–Kleffner syndrome (LKS) 38, 58, 63, 129, 130
learning difficulties 21, 49–50, 65, 100
    management in adolescents 101
    transition to adult epilepsy services 103–4
    see also developmental regression
Lennox–Gastaut syndrome (LGS) 43–4
    management 54, 61, 63
    prognosis 65, 66, 111
levetiracetam
    childhood-onset epilepsies 54, 55
    infantile epilepsies 16
    side effects 118
    status epilepticus 127
liver toxicity 116–17
lumbar puncture 30–1

magnetic resonance imaging (MRI) 3–4
    adolescent-onset epilepsies 84–5
    childhood-onset epilepsies 31, 44
    misinterpretation 140
    pre-surgical 59
magnetic resonance spectroscopy (MRS) 85
male reproductive function 95
mannerisms 35
marijuana use 93–4
Matthews Friends 62
medically refractory epilepsy see intractable epilepsy
medication dispensers 46
medico-legal aspects 139–42
medium chain triglycerides (MCT) 24
meningitis 135

menstruation 94
mental handicap/retardation *see* learning
    difficulties
metabolic disorders 8–9, 22
methylphenidate 50
methylprednisolone 62–3
midazolam
    buccal 115, 126
    intravenous infusion 128
migrating partial seizures in infancy (MPSI)
    13–14, 25, 26
missed doses 46
mitochondrial diseases 88
molecular testing 13
Morrell's procedure (multiple subpial transection)
    61, 130
mortality risks 110, 113
motor behaviors, bizarre 37
movement abnormalities, paroxysmal 35
multiple ligation-dependent probe amplification
    (MLPA) 8
multiple subpial transection (MST) 61, 130
myoclonic–astatic epilepsy (MAE) (Doose
    syndrome) 40, 42–3
    management 61
    prognosis 65, 66
myoclonic epilepsies
    benign, of infancy 15, 27, 111
    juvenile *see* juvenile myoclonic epilepsy
    progressive (PME) 58, 86–8, 96–7
    severe, of infancy *see* Dravet syndrome
myoclonic seizures 5, 12
myoclonus 80, 87

narcolepsy 37
National Institute for Health and Clinical
    Excellence (NICE) 88, 90, 142
neonatal hypoxic–ischemic encephalopathy 20,
    135
neonatal–infantile seizures, benign familial 15
neuro-degenerative disorders 22, 43
neuro-glycopenia 9
neuro-imaging 3–4
    acute seizures 31
    adolescent-onset epilepsies 83
    functional 85
neuronal ceroid lipofuscinosis, juvenile 88
night terrors 35–6, 85
nitrazepam, West syndrome 19
non-epileptic attack disorder (NEAD) 35,
    77–5
non-epileptic paroxysmal disorders 75–9
nurseries 20

obesity 119
oral contraceptive pill 94, 96, 117
oxcarbazepine 55, 95–6

Panayiotopoulos syndrome (early-onset benign
    occipital epilepsy) 41
    management 55
    prognosis 63–4, 111
parasomnias 35–6
paroxysmal disorders, non-epileptic 75–9
partial epilepsies *see* focal epilepsies
partial seizures *see* focal seizures
perioral myoclonia with absences 40
phenobarbital
    in Dravet syndrome 19
    side effects 116, 117–18
phenytoin 22, 89, 97
    side effects 116, 117–18
    status epilepticus 127
photoparoxysmal response (PPR), Dravet
    syndrome 13
photosensitivity 87, 92
piracetam 96–7
polypharmacy 22–3, 46, 89, 97, 138
positron emission tomography (PET) 85
post-traumatic epilepsy (PTE) 135–6
prednisone/prednisolone 17–18, 62–3
pregnancy 54, 81, 94, 117–18
prevention 133–8
    primary and severe familial epilepsies 134
    secondary epilepsies 135–7
    wrong diagnosis 134
    wrong treatment 137–8
progressive myoclonic epilepsies (PME) 58, 86–8,
    96–7
propofol 128, 131
provocative stimuli, avoidance of 92–3
provoked seizures *see* symptomatic seizures
pseudo-epileptic seizures *see* non-epileptic attack
    disorder
psychogenic non-epileptic seizures (PNES)
    see non-epileptic attack disorder
psychological problems 120–1
psychosis 49, 51, 118
psychosocial risks and hazards of epilepsy 119–22
puberty
    effects on established epilepsy 74
    incidence of epilepsy during 73–4, 74
purple hand/glove syndrome 127
pyridoxine dependency 9, 19
pyruvate dehydrogenase complex deficiency 24, 61

quality of life 119–21

rage, paroxysmal 36–7
rashes, drug-induced 116
Rasmussen's syndrome 63, 98, 111, 131
recreational drug use 93–4
recurrence risks
    after AED withdrawal 57, 90, 112–13
    seizures 2, 110–11
reflex anoxic seizures 2, 34, 76
refractory epilepsy *see* intractable epilepsy
regression *see* developmental regression
remission, likelihood of 111–12
restrictions, safety 47–8, 92, 109–10
ring chromosome 20 8
risks and hazards of epilepsy 108–23
    antiepileptic medication 115–19
    minimizing 114–15
    perception and prevention 123
    psychosocial 119–22
    seizure-related 109–14
road traffic accidents, prevention 136
Royal College of Paediatrics and Child Health
    (RCPCH) 89
rufinamide 54

school 78, 121
SCN1A gene mutations 12, 13, 42
SCN1A-related epileptic encephalopathies 12–13
SCN1B gene mutations 42
SCN2A gene mutations 15
SCN2B gene mutations 13
Scottish Intercollegiate Guidelines Network
    (SIGN) 88, 142
seizures
    acute presentation 30–1
    clinical diagnosis 2
    first aid for 114
    first unprovoked 2, 110–11
    inaccurate classification 140
    minor 2
    presentation and differential diagnosis 32
    prolonged, treatment 114–15
    risks and hazards related to 109–14
    symptomatic *see* symptomatic seizures
    triggers 92–5
self-empowerment 102
self-esteem, poor 120
severe myoclonic epilepsy of infancy (SMEI)
    see Dravet syndrome
sexual abuse 78
sexuality 94–5
side effects of antiepileptic drugs 115–19, 138
    assessment 46
    cognitive and behavioral 51, 118–19

dose-related 115–16
idiosyncratic reactions 116–17
in infancy 16, 22
long-term 117
teratogenicity 117–18
weight gain and obesity 119
single photon emission computed tomography
    (SPECT) 85
sleep
    deprivation 93
    disruption 49, 51
    events during 35–6
social growth, limitations to 48
social isolation 101, 122
social outcome, long-term 99–100, 122, 66
sodium valproate *see* valproic acid/sodium
    valproate
sports participation 48
staring episodes 32–3
status epilepticus 126–31
    convulsive (CSE) 126–8
        inappropriate management 141
        management 126–8, 137
        refractory (RCSE) 128
        risks 113–14
    non-convulsive (NCSE) 37, 128–31
        failure to diagnose 140
        treatment to minimize risks 114–15
stereotypies 35
steroid therapy *see* corticosteroid therapy
Stevens–Johnson syndrome 116
stimulant medications 50
stiripentol, in Dravet syndrome 19
stress 93
structural brain lesions 6, 7–8
Sturge–Weber syndrome 24, 98, 111
subacute sclerosing panencephalitis (SSPE) 88
submersion injuries 47, 109
sudden unexpected (or unexplained) death in
    epilepsy (SUDEP) 110, 141
suicide risk 118
sulthiame 55
surgery, epilepsy *see* epilepsy surgery
swimming 47, 109
symptomatic epilepsies 6–9, 44
symptomatic generalized epilepsies
    childhood-onset 53, 54–5, 62–3
    prognosis 65, 66
symptomatic focal (partial) epilepsies
    childhood-onset 53, 55, 61
    prognosis 65, 66
symptomatic seizures
    acute 1, 5, 30

symptomatic seizures (*cont.*)
  in infancy 5, 6
syncope
  cardiogenic 34, 77, 139
  convulsive 75, 76–7
  misdiagnosis as epilepsy 34
  vasovagal 2, 34, 76–7
  versus generalized tonic-clonic seizures 34–5

telomere studies 8
temporal lobe epilepsy/seizures 83–5, 85–6, 136–7
teratogenicity of antiepileptic drugs 54, 81,
      117–18
testosterone, low 95
tetracosactide 17–18, 62–3
thiopentone 128, 131
thought immersion 32
tiagabine 53
Todd's paralysis 111
tongue, bitten 2
tonic seizures 30, 42–3
topiramate
  adolescent-onset epilepsies 81, 89, 95–6
  childhood-onset epilepsies 54
  infantile epilepsies 19
  side effects 118–19
transition to adult epilepsy services 102–4
traumatic brain injury 135–6
triggers, seizure 92–5
trisomy 21 8, 21
tuberous sclerosis
  autism 52
  management 58, 61
  West syndrome 11, 17

Unverricht–Lundborg disease (ULD) 87

vaccinations 20–1
vagal nerve stimulation (VNS) 24, 60, 99
valproic acid/sodium valproate
  adolescent-onset epilepsies 81, 89
  adverse effects 54, 116–17, 117–18
  childhood-onset epilepsies 54, 55
  infantile epilepsies 16, 19
  status epilepticus 127
vasovagal syncope 2, 34, 76–7
video-EEG recordings 78, 97–8
video recordings 6, 29, 77
vigabatrin
  adverse effects 18–19, 117, 118
  West syndrome 17, 18–19, 23
  worsening of epilepsy 53
visual field defects, vigabatrin-induced 18–19, 117
vitamin D supplements 47–8, 94, 117

weight gain 119
West syndrome (WS) 9–12
  autism 52
  cryptogenic or idiopathic 11, 25
  developmental regression 10–11, 21
  epilepsy surgery 24
  ketogenic diet 25
  Lennox–Gastaut syndrome evolving from 43
  prognosis 25–6, 111
  symptomatic 11
  treatment 16, 17–19, 23
Wolf–Hirschhorn syndrome 8

zonisamide 19, 54, 81